Expecting 101: Understanding the Journey Ahead

Kari D. Smith

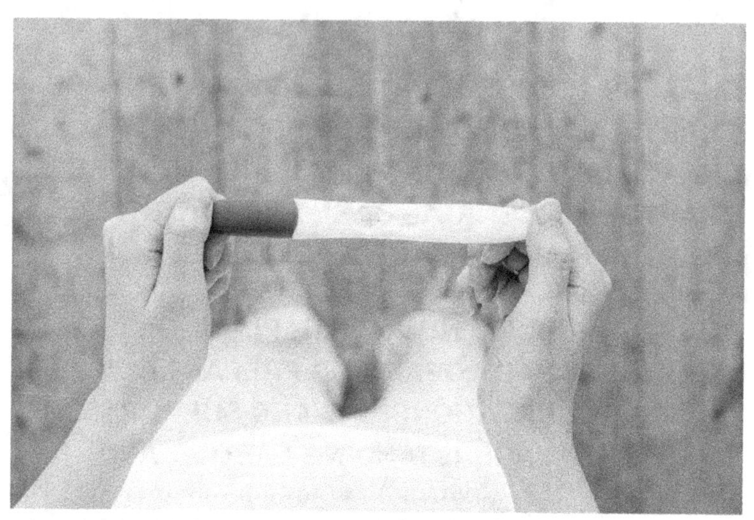

INTRODUCTION

"In the stillness of the night, the soft flutter of a baby's first kick can feel like the thunderous roar of life's most magnificent orchestra. This feeling of a little life stirring inside is a critical moment for many on the road to motherhood. Picture yourself poised on the verge of one of life's greatest experiences, with an expanse of unknowns reaching out before you. What does this quest genuinely entail? How can one prepare for the mysteries of the months ahead?

Welcoming a new life into the world is undoubtedly one of the most profound experiences one can undergo. It is a voyage filled with wonder, obstacles, pleasure, and discovery. Whether you're a first-time expecting parent or re-experiencing the miracle again, each journey is unique and provides its own lessons. With so many sources of information accessible today, it may be hard to wade through the advice, misconceptions, and anecdotes that swirl around pregnancy.

Parenthood is not only a phase; it's an era, a rewriting of everything that we know. I recall the first moment I knew I was going to be a father. My pulse raced as a plethora of feelings flooded over me, from elation to anxiety. That pulse, that flutter, became a sign of a journey that would transform me forever.

Expecting 101: Understanding the Journey Ahead" is aimed at being your valued friend in this changing era. The pages ahead go deep into the numerous dimensions of pregnancy, giving scientific insights, practical assistance, and emotional reassurances. Each chapter is created to help you through the many phases of pregnancy, shining light on what to anticipate and how to best prepare.

Embarking on the route to motherhood may be a rollercoaster of emotions: excitement, fear, pleasure, and trepidation could all intermingle. Our purpose is to provide you with a source of information and consolation and to remind you that although the path could be tough, it is also very rewarding.

So, dear reader, as you stand at the threshold of this wonderful trip, think this: "If the miracle of life can start with just a whisper of a heartbeat, what untold wonders and challenges await as it grows louder and more vibrant?"

We welcome you to flip the page, explore, and discover the marvels and wisdom of expecting. Together, let's comprehend the trip ahead.

Let's begin this adventure together, unraveling the symphony of life and comprehending the voyage ahead.

A. The Miracle of Pregnancy

Pregnancy is a dance of biology and enchantment, a delicate merging of science and awe. The sheer concept that inside a woman's body, a new life might take birth, develop, and finally emerge as a distinct creature is nothing short of astounding. This journey, from the union of a single egg and sperm to the birth of a full person, is an awe-inspiring monument to the strength and majesty of nature.

The miracle starts at conception. Out of millions, one lone sperm successfully unites with an egg to generate what will soon become a zygote. This single cell has the full blueprint for a new human existence, from the color of their eyes to the sound of their laughter. It's a microscopic miracle, the start of a nine-month adventure that will see this small organism turn into a newborn with a beating heart, a dreaming brain, and 10 little fingers and toes.

Throughout gestation, the body's intuition is essential. The womb becomes a shelter, nourishing and safeguarding the developing baby. Around the fifth week, a pulse develops, a rhythmic witness to the life blooming inside. By the conclusion of the first trimester, the fetus has all its organs, muscles, and bones. As the weeks go by, this small creature starts to move, stretch, yawn, and even hiccup.

However, the wonder of pregnancy is not entirely physical. It's also the tremendous emotional and psychological journey a mother experiences. With each passing day, as her body evolves and adapts, a deep and unbreakable link builds. The ambitions, desires, and aspirations she has for her unborn child develop with the infant in her womb.

The climax of this journey, delivery, is a magnificent monument to tenacity, courage, and love. The agony, sweat, and tears experienced throughout labor lead to the incredible pleasure of hearing a baby's first cry, of holding this new life near, and of understanding that two hearts now beat outside but are forever joined.

In essence, pregnancy is a reminder of the deep powers of the human body and the infinite depths of human love. It's a miracle that has been replicated countless times over millennia but stays uniquely special and awe-inspiring with each new life.

B. The Purpose of This Book

In a world abounding with information, views, and advice, particularly concerning pregnancy, there emerges a need for clarity, sincerity, and wisdom. "Expecting 101: Understanding the Journey Ahead" was formed from this precise necessity. While there are innumerable manuals on pregnancy, we intended to build a time that doesn't only educate but also resonates, supports, and empowers its readers.

The major objective of this book is to be a guiding light for individuals on the road to expecting a child. It's a route filled with wonder but also with doubts, questions, and anxieties. This book strives to give answers, debunk misconceptions, and provide comfort. It's intended to reflect the stages of pregnancy, ensuring that as your trip evolves, the book corresponds with your experiences.

But beyond the facts, this book strives to portray the emotional core of pregnancy. We go deep into the emotional, intimate, and spiritual dimensions of being a parent. By sharing tales, observations, and ideas, we hope to make you feel seen, understood, and valued.

Moreover, "Expecting 101" emphasizes that every pregnancy is unique. Hence, rather than prescribing a one-size-fits-all strategy, this book presents a spectrum of experiences, inviting readers to identify their own truths within its pages. It's a book that recognizes the problems but also accentuates the rewards, ensuring that readers feel prepared and motivated.

In essence, the objective of this book is to be a buddy. Whether you're reading it during calm periods of introspection, times of doubt, or spurts of exhilaration, it's here to encourage and guide you. Through understanding, we strive to make the great experience of expecting not only something you endure but something you enjoy, remember, and, above all, celebrate.

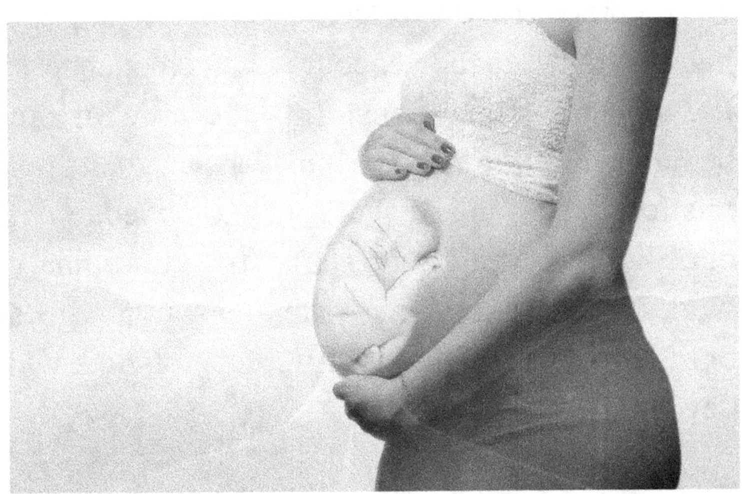

CHAPTER 1: EMBRACING THE NEW ADVENTURE

Every great narrative starts with a step into the unknown. Pregnancy is much like this—a trip into a world full of unfamiliar sensations, emotions, and transforming events. Embracing this new experience is less about preparation and more about submitting to the journey, trusting the process, and relishing the evolving story of becoming a parent.

To embrace is to welcome entirely, and the journey of pregnancy encourages such openness. It's a journey that transforms the core of our being, prompting us to reconsider our goals, our relationships, and even our knowledge of ourselves. As the body starts its extraordinary work of nourishing a new life, the soul too goes on its own path of discovery, contemplation, and development.

The first awareness of expecting a child may be an overpowering combination of emotions: pleasure, fear, excitement, and worry. It's the excitement of the unknown paired with the weight of duty. However, genuinely accepting this trip entails letting go of preconceived beliefs and tight expectations. It's about immersing oneself in the present moment, cherishing the minor milestones, and finding delight in the subtle alterations.

Moreover, accepting this path is also about strengthening resilience. There will be days filled with happiness and others darkened by uncertainties or bodily discomforts. By appreciating both the highs and lows, one may travel this route with grace, compassion, and a sense of humor. Remember, every difficulty overcome and every barrier cleared is a tribute to the strength you never thought you possessed.

Part of this experience is also about creating relationships. With every doctor's appointment, every prenatal class, and every late-night reading session, you're not just accumulating information; you're becoming a member of a community, a tribe of parents and caregivers who have, in their own unique ways, gone on similar journeys. Sharing tales, asking for advice, or just listening may develop friendships that last a lifetime.

In the magnificent tapestry of life, the experience of anticipating is simply a chapter. Yet it's one that leaves an unforgettable impact on the psyche. To embrace this path is to say 'yes' to development, to change, and to love in its purest form. So, when you stand on the edge of this new journey, take a deep breath, believe in the magic of beginnings, and plunge totally into the glorious unknown.

A. The Decision to Start a Family

Decisions dictate our lives' destiny, but few have as much weight and wonder as the decision to create a family. It's a decision that goes beyond the pragmatic, reaching deep into the realms of passion, dedication, and desire. The route to reaching this choice is unique for everyone and impacted by various variables ranging from personal preferences to cultural standards.

For many, the thought of establishing a family isn't a startling discovery but a gradual realization. It's a mosaic of memories and moments: the first time holding a niece or nephew, experiencing the intimate link between parent and kid, or just feeling an innate tug towards parenting. These encounters, sometimes subtle and brief, create the seeds of desire that blossom over time.

Yet, it's not simply about desire. The decision to establish a family frequently entails considerable deliberation. Finances, career paths, health, interpersonal dynamics, and personal preparation all come into play. Discussions turn into meaningful insights, comparing the pleasures of motherhood against the obligations it brings.

For others, cultural and social norms have a crucial impact. The urge to perpetuate family lines or perform perceived tasks might weigh heavily on the decision-making process. However, in current times, many people and couples are rejecting these standards, ensuring that the decision to create a family is both intentional and intensely personal.

There's also an emotional and psychological component. The craving for connection, the urge to nurture, and the desire to share life's highs and lows with a new generation are strong motivators. The thought of experiencing the world again through a child's eyes, of teaching and learning in equal measure, is a magnetic draw for many.

Conversely, the choice may be followed with apprehension. Questions such as "Are we ready?" or "Will I be a good parent?" are typical. These worries, anchored in love and duty, are legitimate and underline the significant implications of the issue at hand.

Ultimately, the choice to create a family is a leap of faith. It's a promise to welcome the unexpected, to love unreservedly, and to develop in ways previously unimagined. Whether the route to this choice is pleasant or difficult, rapid or delayed, it's a monument to the enormous human ability for love, sacrifice, and hope.

B. Emotions and Expectations

The interaction between emotions and expectations is a complicated dance, particularly when it comes to the process of expecting a child. From the first flutter of realization through the expectation of birth, a flurry of sensations envelops a person or couple, typically laced with a tapestry of aspirations, desires, and presumptions about the future.

Emotions in the area of pregnancy are enormous and diverse. The joy of a positive pregnancy test, the wonder of the first ultrasound, the anxiety about health and readiness—all these sensations form a rich emotional landscape. It's a phase characterized by heightened sensitivity, when pleasure is intensified, worries are exaggerated, and even the banal may take on significant meaning.

Tied closely to these feelings are expectations. Every person, consciously or subconsciously, carries images of what pregnancy and motherhood will be like. These are influenced by a plethora of influences: personal upbringing, social conventions, cultural narratives, and even portrayals in the media. We imagine tranquil pregnancies, flawless baby showers, and golden moments of first-time motherhood.

However, reality frequently dances to its own tune. Morning sickness can extend beyond the morning (or the first trimester); the pregnant glow might be followed by episodes of exhaustion; and designing a nursery may not be as uncomplicated as it seems on Pinterest. These differences between anticipation and reality might lead to emotions of disappointment, inadequacy, or skepticism.

Moreover, there's an external factor to consider. Family, friends, and even strangers may have well-intentioned advice or entrenched ideas about pregnancy and parenthood. These external expectations may also contradict personal experiences or wants, creating another layer of emotion to negotiate.

Navigating this delicate weave of emotions and expectations requires patience, communication, and self-awareness. It's crucial to know that it's alright for reality to differ from anticipation. Embracing the unique trip, with all its unexpected twists and turns, is part of the charm.

Open communication, particularly with one's spouse or support network, may give relief. Sharing anxieties, sharing goals, and even venting grievances may lead to moments of clarity and connection. Seeking tales from others who've traveled this journey might also give perspective.

In the end, the dance of emotions and expectations is a rite of passage on the path of expectation. It's a monument to the profundity of the human experience and the tremendous change that awaits. By accepting both the heart's stirrings and the mind's visions, one may discover balance, pleasure, and a greater appreciation for the unfolding journey.

CHAPTER 2: THE SCIENCE OF PREGNANCY

The Science of Pregnancy refers to the various biological processes that occur from conception until birth. This transforming journey entails a sequence of controlled processes that enable a single cell to grow into a full-fledged human newborn. Here's a quick overview:

1. Conception: Pregnancy commences with the fusion of an egg (from the ovary) and a sperm (from the male ejaculation). This fusion culminates in a zygote, a single cell with united genetic material.

2. Cell Division: The zygote starts to divide and proliferate as it moves down the fallopian tube into the uterus, generating a cluster of cells.

3. Implantation: Around a week after conception, the cluster, now termed a blastocyst, attaches itself to the wall of the uterus, signifying the start of the embryonic stage.

4. Hormonal Changes: The implanted blastocyst induces the release of the hormone human chorionic gonadotropin (hCG), leading to maintenance of the corpus luteum and synthesis of progesterone. This ensures the uterus stays appropriate for the developing embryo.

5. Formation of Key Structures:
• Placenta: This organ grows to deliver oxygen and nutrition to the developing baby while eliminating waste.
• Amniotic sac: a fluid-filled sac that covers and cushions the baby during pregnancy.
• Umbilical Cord: connects the fetus to the placenta, allowing for the exchange of nutrients and waste.

6. Fetal Development: The embryo experiences fast development, and by the end of the first trimester, most organs have grown. During the second trimester, the fetus's systems grow and it starts to move. In the third trimester, the fetus further develops and strengthens in preparation for delivery.

7. Birth: Typically at the 40-week mark, hormonal cues induce labor. This includes the dilatation of the cervix, contractions of the uterus, and the final birth of the baby and placenta.

In essence, the Science of Pregnancy digs into the physiological and biochemical changes and processes happening in the mother's body as well as the developmental phases of the fetus, culminating in birth. It's a monument to the exquisite design and flexibility of the human body.

A. Conception and Fertilization

Conception and fertilization are the beginning stages of the wonderful adventure of human development. These two phrases, frequently used interchangeably, describe the first phases of life when new life starts to develop. Let's go deeper into these essential events.

Conception: Conception is the general process in which a sperm cell from a man fertilizes an egg cell from a female, resulting in the creation of a zygote. This process may occur spontaneously inside the female reproductive system or can be assisted outside the body via treatments such as in vitro fertilization (IVF).

The Journey of the Sperm and Egg: During sexual intercourse, a male discharges semen containing millions of sperm into the woman's vagina. These sperm cells go on a tough voyage, swimming past the cervix and into the fallopian tubes. Meanwhile, throughout a woman's monthly menstrual cycle, normally one egg develops and is released from the ovaries in a process called ovulation. This egg then enters the fallopian tube, awaiting possible fertilization.

Fertilization: Fertilization is the exact instant when a single sperm successfully enters the outer layers of the egg. Despite the millions of sperm discharged, only one sperm can and will fertilize the egg. Once a sperm has invaded the egg, the egg instantly undergoes modifications that prevent any additional sperm from entering.

Upon successful entrance, the genetic material (chromosomes) from the sperm mixes with the genetic material from the egg. This fusion results in a zygote, a single cell with a complete set of 46 chromosomes—23 pairs, with one chromosome from each parent in each pair. This zygote holds the genetic blueprint for the formation of a unique human.

The zygote then continues to split and proliferate as it travels down the fallopian tube towards the uterus, laying the groundwork for the following stages of pregnancy.

In essence, conception and fertilization are the amazing processes that signify the birth of human existence. The coming together of two diverse cells to produce a unique individual is a miracle of biology and a tribute to the exquisite design of human reproduction.

B. The Trimesters: A Breakdown

Pregnancy is frequently separated into three different periods known as trimesters. Each trimester is a distinct chapter in the pregnancy, defined by significant changes in both the growing baby and the pregnant mother's body. Let's go into the breakdown of these revolutionary trimesters:

First Trimester: Weeks 1–12
The first trimester represents the beginning of a wonderful adventure. It's at this stage that a fertilized egg transforms from a single cell into a complex organism, with the framework for all major organs set down. The initial indicators of pregnancy, such as missing periods and morning sickness, generally show in this trimester.

• Fetal Development: The embryo develops form, producing a beating heart, rudimentary limbs, and the early stages of facial characteristics.

• Physical Changes: Hormonal fluctuations contribute to changes in the mother's body, including breast soreness, exhaustion, and morning sickness.

• Emotional Landscape: Expectant women may feel a variety of emotions, from happiness to dread, as the reality of pregnancy seeps in.

Second Trimester: Weeks 13–27

Often referred to as the "honeymoon period" of pregnancy, the second trimester gives relief from many first-trimester discomforts. It's a period of enormous growth and development for both the fetus and the mother.

• Fetal Development: Organs grow more, and the fetus starts to move. Facial characteristics grow more pronounced, and its sex may be established by ultrasound.

• Physical Changes: The mother's belly begins to visibly grow, and she may feel the baby's movements, frequently characterized as "fluttering" or "bubbling."
• Emotional Landscape: The first doubts frequently give way to exhilaration as the pregnancy becomes more evident. Expectant parents may begin to connect with their child and make preparations for its birth.

Third Trimester: Weeks 28–40+
The third trimester brings the trip to a close, with the fetus's primary systems completely established and its body focusing on development and maturation. As the due date approaches, anticipation and preparation reach their pinnacle.

• Fetal Development: The baby's organs conclude their development, and it gains weight fast. The lungs continue to grow in preparation for breathing outside the womb.
• Physical Changes: The mother's body continues to adapt, with greater pain due to the

growing growth of the fetus. Braxton Hicks contractions, or "practice contractions," may begin.

• Emotional Landscape: Excitement and anxiety mingle as the reality of approaching fatherhood seeps in. The anticipation of labor and the approaching delivery of the baby become important considerations.

In essence, the trimesters provide a systematic framework for comprehending the extraordinary course of pregnancy. They illustrate the delicate metamorphosis happening inside the mother's body and the amazing growth of the fetus, finally ending in the momentous moment of delivery.

CHAPTER 3: NAVIGATING PHYSICAL CHANGES

"Navigating Physical Changes" often refers to understanding, adjusting to, and controlling the adjustments and transformations our bodies go through during various seasons of life. This may include puberty, pregnancy, postpartum, menopause, age, or even changes due to disease or surgery. Navigating these transitions takes both acceptance and action, ensuring that one's well-being remains a priority.

1. Understanding the Change: Before responding to any change, it's vital to understand its genesis, whether it's hormonal, age-related, or due to particular life experiences. For example, during pregnancy, realizing that weight gain is a normal part of the process might make acceptance easier.

2. Seeking Information: Equip yourself with information about what to anticipate. Whether it's via reading, consulting specialists, or chatting with friends, recognizing what's common helps reduce fears and establish reasonable expectations.

3. Physical Adaptation: Changes could require new routines or habits. For instance, as we age, including strength training may help prevent muscle loss, and during pregnancy, adjusting exercise regimens can guarantee safety for both mother and baby.

4. Emotional Well-Being: Physical changes might have emotional ramifications. For example, postpartum bodily changes could impair a new mother's self-esteem. Recognizing and treating these emotional reactions is key. Seeking help, whether via therapy, support groups, or close friends and family, may be useful.

5. Acceptance and self-love: Every era of life comes with its own distinct set of changes. Embracing them as part of one's ongoing path and practicing self-love and compassion helps produce a positive outlook.

6. Staying Proactive: Regular check-ups, early diagnosis of any anomalies, and proactive health interventions may aid in controlling and reducing unwanted physical changes.

7. Adjusting Lifestyle: Dietary adaptations, workout modifications, skincare regimens, or even outfit changes could be essential as one navigates distinct bodily changes. Being flexible and receptive to these modifications might make the move simpler.

8. Communication: Discussing changes and emotions with loved ones may bring emotional relief and frequently provides a platform to share experiences, ideas, and support.

9. Creating limits: Especially during times like pregnancy or post-surgery, creating limits about one's comfort, relaxation demands, and even subjects of conversation may be vital.

10. Seeking Professional Guidance: Sometimes, addressing bodily changes needs professional assistance. Whether it's a dermatologist for skin changes, a physiotherapist for post-injury rehabilitation, or a counselor for mental upheavals, getting expert support may be helpful.

Navigating bodily changes is a fundamental element of the human experience. While these adjustments may often be painful, they also provide chances for development, resilience, and a greater knowledge of oneself.

A. Changes in the Body

Throughout life, our bodies experience different changes, both subtle and profound. However, few events lead to as many significant bodily alterations as pregnancy. When preparing to sustain and nurture a new life, the body undertakes a sequence of adjustments that are nothing short of amazing.

1. Hormonal Changes: From the time of conception, hormone levels, notably progesterone and human chorionic gonadotropin (hCG), increase to support the growing fetus. These hormones serve a vital function in maintaining the uterine lining for implantation and supporting the placenta and embryonic development.

2. Breast Alterations: Breasts become painful, puffy, and may expand in size. The areolas (the skin covering the nipples) may darken, and tiny glands on the surface could become more apparent. These modifications prepare the breasts for breastfeeding.

3. Cardiovascular System: Blood volume rises to deliver oxygen and nutrients to the fetus, resulting in a higher heart rate. This may occasionally result in palpitations or symptoms of an accelerated heartbeat.

4. Respiratory System: Oxygen consumption rises as the body sustains both the mother and the fetus. This might lead to a sense of shortness of breath or deeper breathing.

5. Musculoskeletal System: As the pregnancy advances, the enlarging uterus may place strain on the spine and pelvis. The body produces a hormone called relaxin, which causes ligaments in the pelvic region to relax and the joints to become looser in preparation for the delivery process. This may occasionally lead to pain or discomfort in the lower back and hips.

6. Skin, Hair, and Nails: Increased blood circulation may contribute to a 'pregnancy glow'. However, some women could develop skin concerns such as increased sensitivity, darkening of the skin (melasma), or acne. Hair may seem fuller, and nails can grow quicker.

7. Digestive Tract: Increased progesterone levels may lead to a relaxed gastrointestinal tract, producing heartburn, constipation, and gas. The enlarging uterus could also impose pressure on the stomach and intestines, adding to similar symptoms.

8. Urinary System: The kidneys work harder during pregnancy to filter the increased blood volume. This leads to more frequent urination. As the baby develops, it may also exert pressure on the bladder, increasing the desire to pee.

9. Immune System: The body modifies its immune response to avoid rejection of the fetus, which is genetically unique. This may render pregnant women more vulnerable to certain infections.

10. Metabolic Changes: Pregnancy boosts the body's metabolic rate, resulting in higher energy needs. There's also a buildup of fat reserves to enable nursing post-delivery.

11. Emotional and cognitive changes: Hormonal fluctuations, bodily discomforts, and the prospect of becoming a parent may contribute to mood swings, anxiety, and changes in sleep habits.

Every woman's experience of these changes is distinct, differing in degree and expression. Nonetheless, these shifts are a tribute to the body's extraordinary power to generate, nourish, and bring forth new life.

B. Common Discomforts and Remedies

Throughout life, and particularly during specialized seasons like pregnancy or aging, our bodies suffer varied discomforts. Recognizing and recognizing these discomforts might aid in obtaining treatment and sustaining well-being. Here's a look at some frequent discomforts and their possible remedies:

1. Heartburn and indigestion:

• Remedies: eating smaller, more frequent meals; avoiding spicy, acidic, and oily foods; remaining upright after meals; over-the-counter antacids (always speak with a healthcare expert).

2. Constipation:

• Remedies: increasing fiber intake via fruits, vegetables, and whole grains; drinking enough water; regular exercise; over-the-counter stool softeners; or fiber supplements after visiting a healthcare expert.

3. Headaches:

• Remedies: adequate rest; stress-relief strategies like meditation or deep breathing exercises; keeping a regular eating schedule; avoiding recognized triggers; over-the-counter pain remedies; but always consult before using any drugs.

4. Nausea or morning sickness:

• Remedies: Eating dry toast or crackers before waking up; ingesting ginger tea or ginger candies; avoiding strong scents; acupressure bracelets; vitamin B6 supplements (with a doctor's permission).

5. Back discomfort:

• Remedies: maintaining excellent posture; utilizing a firm mattress; wearing supportive shoes; hot or cold packs; prenatal massages; exercises or stretches suited for back discomfort.

6. Leg Cramps:

• Remedies: Gentle leg stretches; ensuring appropriate calcium and magnesium intake; keeping hydrated; avoiding sitting or standing for lengthy periods

7. Nasal Congestion:

• Remedies: saline nasal sprays; humidifiers or vaporizers; elevating the head when sleeping.

8. Hemorrhoids:

• Remedies: over-the-counter lotions or ointments; witch hazel pads; warm sitz baths; increasing fiber intake.

9. Fatigue:
• Remedies: adequate sleep and rest; short naps throughout the day; remaining active with modest activities; maintaining a balanced diet.

10. Swelling of Ankles and Feet:
• Remedies: elevating feet when feasible; avoiding tight shoes or socks; keeping hydrated; wearing supportive footwear.

11. Insomnia:
• Remedies: Establishing a regular sleep routine; providing a peaceful and dark sleeping environment; avoiding coffee or heavy meals before bed; using relaxing methods like deep breathing or gentle stretching.

12. Mood Swings:
• Remedies: regular exercise; appropriate sleep; joining support groups; counseling or therapy; communicating emotions with loved ones.

It's important to remember that although these cures might bring comfort, they aren't universal answers. Individual responses might vary, and any persistent or severe pain should be handled by a healthcare expert. Furthermore, before using any drug or supplement, it's vital to contact a doctor to guarantee safety, particularly during periods like pregnancy.

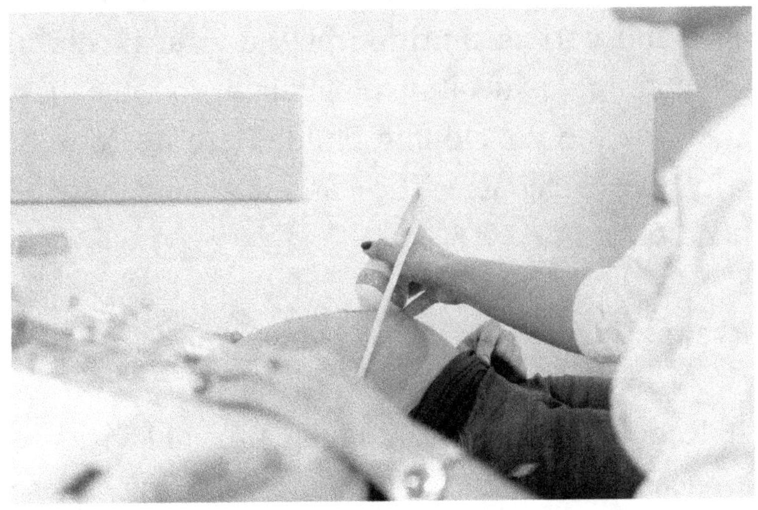

CHAPTER 4: PRENATAL CARE AND NUTRITION

During pregnancy, taking care of both the mother's health and the growing baby's well-being is of the utmost significance. Prenatal care and correct nutrition play a critical role in maintaining a healthy pregnancy and the best start for the developing child. Here's a look at why these characteristics are vital and how to handle them:

Prenatal Care:

1. Regular check-ups: Regular prenatal visits to a healthcare practitioner are crucial. These sessions monitor the baby's progress, identify any possible issues, and ensure the mother's health is on track.

2. Screenings and Tests: Prenatal care involves numerous screenings and tests, such as blood

tests, ultrasounds, and genetic screenings, to monitor the baby's health and growth.

3. Nutritional counseling: Healthcare practitioners give counseling on optimal weight growth, dietary needs, and supplements, ensuring both the mother and infant obtain important nutrients.

4. Exercise and Activity: Staying active throughout pregnancy may help control weight gain, increase mood, and improve circulation. However, it's crucial to contact a healthcare physician before beginning or maintaining any workout regimen.

5. Managing Discomforts: Prenatal care covers typical discomforts, including nausea, back pain, and exhaustion, and gives techniques for alleviation.

Prenatal Nutrition:

1. Balanced Diet: A well-rounded diet contains a range of fruits, vegetables, whole grains, lean meats, and dairy products. Focus on eating nutrient-dense meals that supply vitamins, minerals, and other important nutrients.

2. Folic Acid: Adequate folic acid consumption during early pregnancy lessens the incidence of birth abnormalities. Leafy greens, fortified cereals, and legumes are excellent sources.

3. Iron: Iron promotes increasing blood volume during pregnancy. Include lean meats, legumes, and fortified cereals to avoid anemia.

4. Calcium: Calcium assists in the baby's bone formation. Dairy products, fortified plant-based milk, and leafy greens are calcium-rich options.

5. Protein: Protein fosters the development of tissues and cells. Incorporate lean meats, poultry, fish, eggs, dairy products, and plant-based protein sources.

6. Omega-3 Fatty Acids: These are vital for prenatal brain and eye development. Include fatty fish (with low mercury levels) or try omega-3 supplements.

7. Hydration: Staying well-hydrated is vital for maintaining amniotic fluid levels and sustaining the increasing blood volume.

8. Limit Caffeine and Avoid Harmful Substances: Limit caffeine consumption and avoid alcohol, smoking, and recreational drugs since these may damage the growing infant.

9. Consultation: Every pregnancy is unique. Consult a healthcare physician or a trained dietitian to customize nutrition recommendations to individual requirements, particularly if there are specific health concerns or dietary limitations.

10. Adequate Calories: Pregnancy needs increased calories, particularly in the second and

third trimesters. Focus on nutrient-dense meals to fulfill increased energy demands.

Prenatal care and nutrition are pillars of a healthy pregnancy. They supply the critical building blocks for the baby's growth and assist the mother's well-being during this transforming journey.

A. Choosing a Healthcare Provider

Selecting the correct healthcare professional is a major choice, particularly during transformative times like pregnancy or while coping with chronic diseases. The decision may impact one's entire health experience, the quality of treatment received, and peace of mind. Here are the stages and factors to guide this critical decision:

1. Identify Your Needs:
• Determine what you're searching for. Do you need a specialist or a general practitioner? If

45

you're pregnant, are you contemplating an obstetrician, a family physician who delivers babies, or a midwife?

2. Research and referrals:
• Ask friends, relatives, or coworkers for referrals.
• Check internet reviews and ratings, but approach them with an open mind.
• Consult professional organizations or medical societies that give names of qualified professionals in different disciplines.

3. Check credentials:
• Ensure the practitioner is board-certified in their specialty.
• Investigate whether there are any prior malpractice claims or disciplinary measures against them.

4. Consider expertise:
• For certain problems or treatments, it might be helpful to know your practitioner has substantial expertise in that area.

5. Hospital or Clinic Affiliation:
• If it's necessary for you to deliver or be treated at a certain hospital, check that your selected practitioner has privileges there.

6. Communication approach:
• It's crucial to feel comfortable with your provider's communication approach. Do they listen to your concerns? Do they explain things in a manner you understand?

7. Gender Preference:
• For certain people, the gender of the healthcare professional may be a key factor, particularly for treatments connected to reproductive or sexual health.

8. Location and Accessibility:
• Consider the provider's office location. Is it readily accessible? Is there parking available? How about public transit links?
Check their office hours. Do they coincide with your schedule?

9. Technological Savviness:

• In today's digital world, people appreciate physicians that employ electronic health records, provide telemedicine treatments, or communicate via secure web portals.

10. Insurance and Financial Considerations:

• Ensure the provider accepts your health insurance.

• Understand any out-of-pocket charges you could incur.

11. Initial Consultation:

• Consider organizing a "get-to-know-you" appointment. This might give you a sense of the provider's style, the workplace setting, and the support team.

12. Trust Your Instincts:

• Sometimes, the greatest indicator is your intuition. Do you feel comfortable, respected, and heard?

In essence, selecting a healthcare provider is a personal choice affected by distinct requirements and interests. It's important to spend time making an educated decision since a trustworthy healthcare connection may substantially improve one's health journey.

B. The Importance of a Healthy Diet

A nutritious diet is crucial to our well-being, functioning as the fundamental pillar that supports both our physical and mental health. Here's a look at why a well-balanced diet is necessary and the many advantages it offers:

1. Supports Growth and Development:
• From the early stages of life, a healthy diet encourages optimal growth and development, which is particularly crucial throughout childhood and adolescence when bones,

muscles, and cognitive capacities are rapidly growing.

2. Boosts Immunity:

• A diet rich in vitamins, minerals, and antioxidants improves the immune system, making it more efficient in warding off infections and disorders.

3. Maintains a Healthy Weight:

• A balanced diet, along with regular physical exercise, helps maintain body weight, minimizing the risk of obesity and related health conditions, including type 2 diabetes and cardiovascular illnesses.

4. Promotes Cardiovascular Health:

• Consuming heart-healthy foods, including whole grains, fruits, vegetables, lean meats, and omega-3 fatty acids, helps lessen the risk of heart illnesses and maintain healthy blood pressure levels.

5. Optimizes Brain Health:

• Nutrients including omega-3 fatty acids, antioxidants, and certain vitamins are associated with increased cognitive function, improved concentration, and a lower risk of neurodegenerative illnesses.

6. Aids Digestion:

• Dietary fiber, found in fruits, vegetables, and whole grains, aids normal digestion and maintains a healthy gut, minimizing concerns like constipation or irritable bowel syndrome.

7. Regulates Blood Sugar:

• A nutritious diet helps regulate blood sugar levels, minimizing the risk of type 2 diabetes and maintaining continuous energy throughout the day.

8. Supports Bone Health:

• Nutrients like calcium and vitamin D, found in dairy products and fortified diets, are crucial for keeping healthy bones and teeth.

9. Enhances mood and mental well-being:

• Certain meals may impact neurotransmitter function, possibly influencing mood. For instance, the amino acid tryptophan, present in turkey and nuts, may stimulate serotonin synthesis, frequently nicknamed the "feel-good" hormone.

10. Prevents chronic illnesses:

• A balanced diet decreases the risk of several chronic illnesses, including hypertension, stroke, heart disorders, some malignancies, and osteoporosis.

11. Promotes Skin Health:

• Hydration, together with vitamins and minerals from a balanced diet, may contribute to beautiful skin, minimizing indications of aging and skin problems.

12. Ensures Longevity:

• Several studies show that a diet rich in fruits, vegetables, whole grains, and lean meats will improve longevity and offer a higher quality of life.

In essence, the dietary choices we make every day directly influence our entire health and well-being. Adopting a healthy diet isn't just about limiting calories or remaining skinny; it's about feeding the body, boosting life quality, and building the basis for a healthier future.

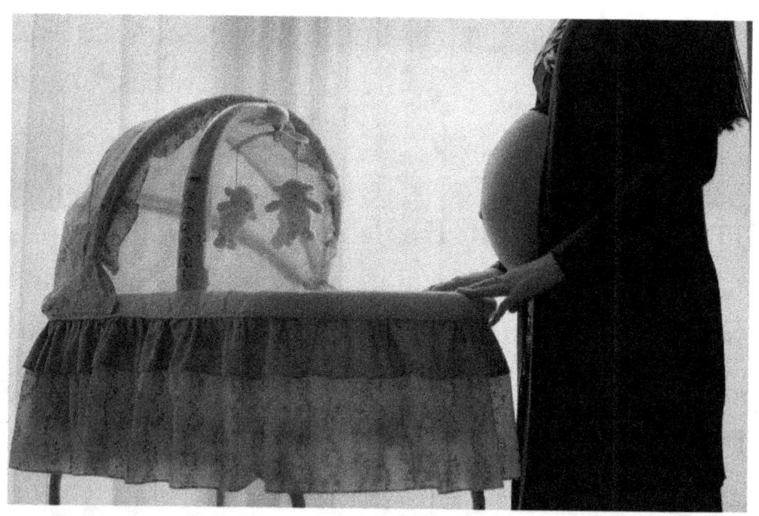

CHAPTER 5: MENTAL AND EMOTIONAL WELL-BEING

Mental and emotional well-being is as vital as physical health, playing a critical role in our overall quality of life. It includes our capacity to control thoughts, emotions, and actions, deal with problems, and develop good relationships. Let's investigate its relevance and the variables impacting it

1. Definition:
• Mental and emotional well-being refers to a condition where people realize their strengths, handle life's stressors, work successfully, and make significant contributions to their communities.

2. Influence on Daily Activities:
• Our mental and emotional condition determines how we manage stress, react to people, and make decisions. A pleasant sense of

well-being increases productivity, creativity, and interpersonal connections.

3. Resilience Against Challenges:

• Strong mental and emotional health helps people bounce back from adversities, setbacks, and traumas, perceiving them as temporary challenges rather than insurmountable obstacles.

4. Influence on Physical Health:

• Mental well-being directly affects physical health. Chronic stress, despair, or anxiety may lead to significant physical health consequences, including heart disease, high blood pressure, or a compromised immune system.

5. Developing healthy relationships:

• Emotional intelligence and well-being create understanding, empathy, and effective communication, all of which are crucial for developing and sustaining healthy relationships.

6. Key Components:

• Self-awareness: recognizing and comprehending one's feelings, strengths, limitations, desires, and values.
• Self-regulation: managing disruptive emotions and impulses efficiently.
• Motivation: Being motivated to succeed for the sake of achieving.
• Empathy: recognizing and comprehending the feelings of others
• Social Skills: Handling relationships, developing networks, and navigating social complexity

7. Maintaining Mental and Emotional Well-Being:

• Healthy Lifestyle Choices: Regular physical exercise and a balanced diet may increase mood and mental well-being.
• Stress Management: Techniques like meditation, deep breathing exercises, and journaling may help manage and decrease stress.
• Sleep: Adequate sleep rejuvenates the mind and body, enhancing mood, cognition, and stress resistance.

• Connecting with Others: Building and sustaining good personal connections gives emotional support and enhances life experiences.
• Creating Boundaries: Knowing one's limitations and creating good boundaries with one's job, relationships, and hobbies may help avoid burnout.

8. Seeking Help:
• Recognizing when professional aid is required is a show of strength. Therapists, counselors, and other mental health experts may offer ways to promote mental and emotional well-being.

In essence, mental and emotional well-being is a vital element of our overall health. Prioritizing and nourishing it is not a luxury but a requirement for a healthy, fulfilled, and meaningful existence.

A. Coping with Hormonal Shifts

Hormones serve a critical function in regulating several physiological processes in our bodies. However, throughout various life periods or owing to certain situations, hormonal imbalances may emerge, leading to a cascade of physical and mental changes. Understanding and efficiently managing these alterations helps lessen their influence on everyday life. Here's how:

1. Awareness and Education:
• Understand the fundamental reasons Hormonal alterations may come from normal life events (puberty, pregnancy, menopause), medical diseases (thyroid disorders, diabetes, PCOS), or even certain drugs.

2. Monitoring Symptoms:
• Keeping a diary may help document symptoms associated with hormone imbalances, such as mood swings, sleep problems, hunger changes, or menstruation abnormalities. This may be

valuable for both self-awareness and interactions with healthcare practitioners.

3. Dietary Choices:
• Certain foods may alter hormone production. For instance, taking omega-3 fatty acids, found in fish and flaxseeds, may help control hormone levels. Minimizing sugar and processed meals helps balance insulin and other hormones.

4. Regular Exercise:
• Physical exercise assists in controlling hormones like insulin, adrenaline, and cortisol. It may also stimulate mood-enhancing chemicals like endorphins.

5. Stress Management:
• Chronic stress may worsen hormonal abnormalities, notably cortisol. Techniques like meditation, deep breathing, yoga, and regular relaxation may help reduce stress.

6. Adequate Sleep:

• Hormones controlling stress, hunger, and growth are regulated by sleep. Ensure a regular sleep pattern and establish a peaceful atmosphere to promote hormonal balance.

7. Limit stimulants:

• Excessive coffee or alcohol might alter hormonal balance. It's suggested that you take them in moderation.

8. Seek Medical Guidance:

• Consultation with healthcare specialists, such as endocrinologists or gynecologists, may give clarification on hormone irregularities. They may propose treatments, therapies, or lifestyle modifications customized to individual requirements.

9. Hormone Replacement Therapy (HRT):

• For some, particularly those undergoing menopause or specific medical issues, HRT could be prescribed. This therapy includes taking synthetic hormones to offset deficits. However, it's vital to examine the advantages and hazards with a medical specialist.

10. Alternative Therapies:

• Some people get relief from symptoms of hormone imbalance via acupuncture, herbal medicines, or supplements. Always contact a healthcare practitioner before initiating any alternative therapy.

11. Emotional Support:

• Hormonal fluctuations may influence mood and emotional well-being. Talking to friends, relatives, or support groups may bring understanding and comfort. Professional counseling or therapy may also teach coping skills.

12. Stay Updated:

• Hormonal therapy and knowledge change with research. Staying updated on the newest research or therapies might provide further alternatives for regulating hormonal changes.

In conclusion, although hormonal shifts may be stressful, recognizing their sources, appreciating their influence, and applying efficient coping skills can substantially simplify the trip while maintaining physical and mental stability.

B. Communicating with Your Partner

Effective communication is the cornerstone of every successful relationship. Open, honest, and compassionate discussion creates understanding, builds trust, and enhances the link between couples. Here's a guide on how to improve communication with your partner:

1. Active Listening:
• Give your complete attention while your companion talks. Avoid interrupting and truly attempt to comprehend their position. Sometimes, just being heard may be tremendously affirming.

2. Use "I" Statements:

• Instead of expressing, "You never listen to me," go for "I feel unheard when... This strategy exposes sentiments without placing blame, lowering the risk of defensiveness.

3. Avoid accusations:

• Accusing or assigning blame might make your spouse defensive. Aim for a discourse that seeks understanding rather than pointing fingers.

4. Stay Calm:

• Heated debates may develop rapidly. If emotions run too high, take a break and return to the topic when both of you are calmer.

5. Be Honest:

• Openness develops trust. Even though the truth is difficult, honesty builds true connection and understanding.

6. Choose the Right Time:

• Addressing serious problems while one or both of you are tired, anxious, or preoccupied isn't beneficial. Find a moment when both of you are calm and can concentrate on the chat.

7. Non-verbal Communication:

• Be conscious of your body language. Often, non-verbal clues like facial expressions or posture transmit more than words.

8. Ask Open-ended Questions:

• Instead of asking questions that may be answered with a simple "yes" or "no," use open-ended ones like "How did that make you feel?" to stimulate deeper discourse.

9. Compromise:

• A partnership comprises two people with separate opinions and emotions. Finding a middle ground demonstrates respect for both sides.

10. Express Appreciation:

• Regularly recognize and thank your spouse. Expressing thanks and emphasizing positive traits helps create goodwill.

11. Seek Outside Help:
• If communication hurdles remain, seek couples therapy. A professional may provide tools and tactics to promote discussion and understanding.

12. Practice Empathy:
• Put yourself in your partner's shoes. Empathetic understanding may overcome numerous communication obstacles.

13. Revisit Past Conversations:
• Periodically checking in on earlier talks or concerns ensures that both partners feel noticed and understood, and it helps measure the growth of the relationship.

14. Establish limits:
• Clearly identify personal limits in terms of space, time, and emotional demands. Respecting

these restrictions demonstrates compassion and understanding.

In essence, good communication in your relationship entails mutual respect, understanding, and an ongoing effort to overcome gaps. It's a dynamic process that, when encouraged, may lead to a deep and rewarding relationship.

CHAPTER 6: BUILDING A BIRTH PLAN

A birth plan is a document that expresses your preferences and desires for birth to your healthcare team. While it's vital to be flexible since births may be unexpected, a plan helps guide the process and ensure your goals are recognized. Here's how to construct a detailed birth plan:

1. Research and Education:
• Familiarize yourself with different delivery methods, interventions, and pain treatment

alternatives. Consider taking birthing courses to obtain insights.

2. Environment:
• Decide where you'd want to give birth: a hospital, a birthing facility, or at home.
• Consider the ambiance: Do you want dimmed lights, certain music, or any particular aromas?

3. Labor Preferences:
• Position and Mobility: Indicate whether you wish to move around, utilize birthing balls, or adopt various positions throughout labor.
• Monitoring: Specify whether you'd want continuous electronic fetal monitoring or if you're okay with intermittent monitoring.
• Pain reduction: state whether you'd want natural pain reduction options, such as massage or a warm bath, or medical interventions like an epidural.

4. Birth Companions:

• Identify someone you'd want to be there throughout labor and delivery, such as your spouse, a doula, or a close friend.

5. Interventions:

• Express your choices for medical interventions such as membrane rupture, the use of Pitocin to initiate or augment labor, or vacuum extraction.

6. Delivery Preferences:

• Position: Do you have a preferred position for delivery?

• Cord Clamping: Specify whether you'd like quick clamping of the umbilical cord or if you'd like delayed clamping.

• Skin-to-Skin Contact: Mention whether you prefer to have immediate skin-to-skin contact with your baby following delivery.

7. C-Section Preferences:

• In case a cesarean becomes required, establish your desires. For instance, you could prefer a transparent drape to watch the birth or to have direct skin-to-skin contact post-delivery.

8. After Delivery:

• Specify your preferences for the baby's first hours. Do you desire immediate breastfeeding? Do you have preferences about normal treatments like eye ointment or vitamin K shots?

9. Feeding:

• Indicate whether you want to breastfeed, formula feed, or a mix of both.

10. Special Considerations:

• Mention any unique cultural or religious rituals you'd wish observed or any other specific requirements.

11. Plan for Unexpected Scenarios:

• Consider discussing and recording your wishes in case of unexpected results, including if the baby has to be in the NICU.

12. Review and Discuss:

• Share your birth plan with your healthcare practitioner. They may give comments, explain hospital regulations, and verify that your goals fit with what's medically viable.

13. Stay Flexible:
• Childbirth may be unexpected. Use the birth plan as a guide, but stay open to adjustments if they're in the best interest of you or your baby.

Lastly, consider taking extra copies of your birth plan to the hospital or birthing facility. This ensures that the attending team is aware of your choices, resulting in a more customized delivery experience.

A. Hospital vs. Home Birth

Choosing the setting in which to give birth is a very personal choice. Both hospital and home deliveries have their benefits and concerns. Here's a comparison to help pregnant parents make an educated choice:

Hospital Birth Advantages:

1. Medical Resources: Hospitals are equipped with modern medical equipment and people to treat emergencies or difficulties.

2. Pain Management: Options like epidurals or specialized drugs are accessible exclusively in a hospital environment.

3. Staff Availability: Obstetricians, anesthesiologists, pediatricians, and nurses are on-site and available.

4. Neonatal Care: If the infant requires urgent specialist care, neonatal intensive care units (NICU) are often offered in bigger hospitals.

Considerations:
1. Clinical Environment: Some individuals find hospitals to be impersonal or scary, which may impair their delivery experience.

2. Intervention Rates: There may be a greater possibility of medical interventions, including

cesarean sections or labor inductions, in a hospital environment.

3. Hospital regulations: Certain hospital regulations could restrict movement during labor or regulate other parts of the delivery process.

4. Infection Risk: While hospitals maintain stringent cleaning standards, they are also locations where ill people gather, which can offer a (usually modest) risk of infection.

Home Birth Advantages:

1. Familiar Environment: Being in a familiar and comfortable location might help some women relax, perhaps helping the course of labor.

2. Personalized Experience: Home births can provide for a more personalized labor and delivery experience.

3. Adjusting the Atmosphere: The mother has the freedom to adjust aspects like lighting, music, the presence of people, and other ambiance-related characteristics.

4. Fewer Medical Interventions: Home births often entail fewer medical interventions, resulting in a more natural childbirth experience.

Considerations:

1. Emergency Situations: If issues emerge, the essential medical equipment or staff may not be readily accessible. A transfer to a hospital might be necessary, which takes time.

2. Limited Pain Management: Medical pain treatment alternatives, including epidurals, are not accessible with home deliveries.

3. Insurance Considerations: Not all insurance plans support home births or could only cover

select components, resulting in significant out-of-pocket payments.

4. Professional Assistance: It's vital to have a competent midwife or healthcare expert present during a home delivery. Ensure they have the relevant certificates and experience.

Before picking, it's vital to examine issues including the pregnancy's risk level, distance from a hospital, personal comfort, and the availability of qualified delivery attendants for home births. It's also important to explore choices with healthcare experts since they may give insights based on individual health and circumstances. Regardless of the decision, the emphasis is on the safety and well-being of both the mother and the infant.

B. Exploring Pain Management Options

Pain management during labor and delivery is a key issue for many pregnant women. There are different methods accessible, ranging from medicinal procedures to natural approaches. Here's an outline of typical pain treatment strategies to consider:

Medical Interventions:

1. Epidural:
• This is a localized anesthetic delivered by an injection in the spine, numbing the lower half of the body. It's good for pain relief, yet it enables the mother to remain awake and aware.

2. Spinal Block:
• Similar to an epidural, except it's a one-time injection that delivers immediate and intense pain relief for a shorter duration. Often used during cesarean sections.

3. Combined Spinal-Epidural (CSE):
This combines the advantages of both the epidural and spinal blocks.

4. Narcotics:
Medications like morphine or fentanyl may be delivered intravenously or intramuscularly. They don't remove pain but may diminish it.

5. Nitrous Oxide:
Inhaled via a mask, this gas may help relieve pain and anxiety. It's less strong than an epidural or drugs.

6. Pudendal Block:
• An anesthetic inserted into the vaginal wall to numb the perineum during the pushing stage or for episiotomy

Natural Pain Management Techniques:

1. Breathing Techniques:
• Focused and structured breathing helps distract from contractions and aid in oxygenating the body.

2. Hydrotherapy:

• Immersing in a warm bath or shower may help relax muscles and give pain relief.

3. Massage:
• Gentle massage, particularly on the lower back, may release stress and lessen discomfort.

4. Movement and Position Changes:
• Walking, swaying, rocking, or changing postures may assist in dealing with contractions and could even help in advancing labor.

5. Counterpressure:
• Applying pressure on the lower back during contractions might bring relief.

6. Acupressure and Reflexology:
• Applying pressure to certain spots on the body may trigger natural pain alleviation systems.

7. Visualization and Distraction:
• Focusing on pleasant thoughts or pictures might distract from the discomfort. Listening to music or viewing a movie could also assist.

8. Warm or cold compression:
• Applying warmth helps relax stiff muscles, while cold can numb regions of pain.

9. Doula Support:
• A doula offers emotional support, comfort methods, and advocacy, which may improve the whole delivery experience and assist with pain management.

10. TENS (Transcutaneous Electrical Nerve Stimulation):
• A device gives moderate electrical impulses to the back, lowering pain signals to the brain.

Things to Consider:
• Personal Preference: Some women want to experience birth without medical treatments, while others emphasize pharmacological pain relief.
• Health and Safety: Discuss choices with your healthcare professional, evaluating any possible dangers or problems.

Flexibility:

• Labor may be unpredictable. While it's beneficial to have a plan, be open to changes based on the situation.

Ultimately, the choice of pain management should align with the mother's comfort, her health conditions, and the medical team's recommendations, ensuring the safety and well-being of both the mother and the baby.

CHAPTER 7: BABY GEAR AND PREPARATION

Welcoming a new baby includes an amalgamation of feelings, from excitement and delight to the overwhelming reality of the preparations necessary. Having the correct baby gear not only assures your kid's comfort but also simplifies parental responsibilities. Here's a curated list of crucial infant gear and preparatory tips:

Essential Baby Gear

1. Sleep Essentials

• Crib or bassinet: choose one that corresponds to current safety regulations.
• Mattress and waterproof covers: ensure a close fit to avoid gaps.
• Sleep sacks: safer than blankets for keeping infants warm.

2. Feeding Necessities

• Breast Pump and Accessories: helpful if you're going to breastfeed and save milk.
• Bottles and Sterilizer: Opt for anti-colic bottles first.
• High Chair: for when the infant begins eating food, around the 6-month mark.

3. Diapering

• Diapers: Stock both cloth and disposable versions to determine what works best.
• Changing Pad or Table: A safe area to change diapers
• Wipes and diaper rash cream: essentials for each changing session

4. Clothing

• Bodysuits: Zippered ones are more handy than buttoned ones.

• Soft caps and mittens: protect infants from the cold and from scratching themselves.

• Swaddling Cloths: Many newborns sleep better when swaddled.

5. On-the-Go

• Car Seat: Invest in a decent-quality, rear-facing car seat.

• Stroller: Depending on your lifestyle, you could desire a daily, jogging, or travel stroller.

• Baby Carrier: Enables hands-free carrying, fostering bonding.

6. Bathing and grooming

• Infant Bathtub: Some come with a sling for infants.

• Gentle Baby Shampoo and Body Wash: Fragrance-free is frequently preferable for delicate skin.

• Baby Nail Clippers: Babies' nails grow rapidly and may be sharp.

7. Entertainment and development
• Play mat or gym: great for tummy time and sensory exploration.
• Swing or bouncer: useful for amusing or relaxing the infant.
• Soft toys and rattles: ensure they are safe for chewing and don't have little removable components.

8. Health and safety
• Digital Thermometer: To check a baby's temperature • First-Aid Kit: Stocked with baby-safe products
• Baby Monitor: This is especially beneficial if the baby's room is separate from yours.

Preparation Tips

1. Create a Functional Nursery: Organize the nursery in such a manner that the basics are within arm's reach, particularly near the changing table and cot.

2. Pre-wash baby clothing: Use a light detergent to wash all baby clothing, blankets, and linens before use.

3. Setup a Feeding Station: Whether you're nursing or formula-feeding, have a comfy space with vital supplies like burp cloths, a water bottle, and snacks.

4. Install the car seat early: Get the car seat fitted and tested at a local inspection station before the infant comes.

5. Pack a Hospital Bag: Prepare a bag with materials you'll need for the hospital stay, including clothing for you and the baby, necessities, and any documents.

Remember, although the market is saturated with a range of infant supplies, it's crucial to discriminate between what's touted as a "must-have" and what's actually required for your individual scenario. Prioritize safety, comfort, and usefulness while buying things for your infant.

A. Creating a Comfortable Nursery

Designing a nursery goes beyond aesthetics; it's about establishing a pleasant, practical place that caters to both the baby's and parents' requirements. Here's a guide to guaranteeing the nursery you put up is comfortable, secure, and inviting:

1. Start with the basics
• Crib: Ensure it fulfills the newest safety regulations. Avoid drop-side cribs and go for one with an adjustable mattress height.
• Changing Table: A safe area to change diapers, especially with storage choices for supplies.
• Dresser: for storing baby clothing, blankets, and other needs.

• A comfortable chair is essential for feeding and soothing the infant. Consider a glider or a soft, cushioned recliner.

2. Choose a soothing color palette
• Soft, subdued hues or pastels may have a soothing impact. Consider colors of light blue, gentle greens, creamy whites, or delicate pinks and purples.

3. Prioritize safety
• Anchor Furniture: Secure dressers and other heavy furniture to the wall to prevent them from tipping.
• Cordless Window Treatments: Opt for cordless blinds or curtains to prevent choking dangers.
• Outlet Covers: Secure any accessible outlets with safety covers.
• Avoid placing the crib near windows. This decreases the chance of drafts and ensures cables or curtain ties are out of reach.

4. Consider lighting

• Soft Lighting: Use dimmable lights or install a dimmer switch. Soft illumination is perfect for overnight diaper changes or feedings without being too bright for the infant.

• Blackout curtains: These help darken the room, promoting greater sleep during nap times.

5. Organize efficiently

• Use boxes, baskets, and dividers to arrange baby clothing, diapers, and other supplies. Labeling may be beneficial.

• Keep commonly used products, like diapers and wipes, within easy reach.

6. Incorporate Soothing Sounds:

• Consider adding a white noise machine or a sound system to play lullabies. Consistent, gentle tones help calm newborns and cover household disturbances.

7. Personalize the Space:

• Incorporate objects that give the nursery a personal touch—family pictures, a treasured blanket, or wall decals with beloved quotations or figures.

8. Add Textures for Comfort:
• Incorporate soft rugs (if you have hard flooring), velvety blankets, and soft cushions (for decorating reasons; avoid putting them in the crib).

9. Create a Reading Corner:
• A tiny bookshelf loaded with colorful baby books, along with a nice floor cushion, may inculcate the habit of reading from an early age.

10. Ensure Proper Ventilation and Temperature:
• Use a baby-friendly fan or an air purifier to circulate air. The optimal nursery temperature is between 68°F and 72°F (20°C to 22°C).

11. Opt for washable materials.
• Spills and mishaps are unavoidable. Wherever feasible, utilize washable materials for simpler cleaning.

Remember, the nursery is an area where many first memories are established, from midnight feedings to daytime playtimes. While it's crucial for it to be practical and secure, it should also be an expression of love, care, and the excitement of new beginnings.

B. Must-Have Baby Essentials

When preparing for a new baby, it may be stressful to discern what's genuinely vital. Here's a quick list of must-have goods to guarantee you're well-prepared for your little one's arrival:

1. Sleeping Essentials
• Crib or bassinet: ensure it meets safety regulations.
• Crib Mattress and Protective Cover: The mattress should fit snugly inside the crib.
• Sleep sacks or swaddle blankets are safer than loose blankets and may help newborns sleep more peacefully.

2. Feeding Necessities:

• Breast Pump: If nursing, a pump may help sustain milk supply and enable others to feed the infant.

• Bottles: Even for nursing parents, having a few bottles is beneficial.

• Sterilizer: ensures bottles, nipples, and other feeding items are germ-free.

• Formula: For mothers who prefer to formula-feed or want it as a backup.

• Burp Cloths: Essential for feedings to capture any spit-ups

3. Diapering Basics

• Diapers: Stock up on both cloth and disposable versions.

• Wipes: Fragrance-free varieties are pleasant on babies skin.

• Changing Pad: Provides a comfortable location for diaper changes.

• Diaper Rash Cream: Helps prevent and cure diaper rashes.

• Diaper Bag: For organizing and carrying all infant needs while on the road.

4. Clothing

• Onesies: both short-sleeved and long-sleeved, depending on the season.

• Sleepers or pajamas: for comfy evening wear

• Hats: useful for keeping babies' heads warm.

• Socks or boots: Even for newborns born in warmer areas, a few pairs are required.

5. Bath Time

• Infant Bathtub: This can make washing a wriggly infant simpler and safer.

• Baby Shampoo and Body Wash: Tear-free and gentle formulas are recommended.

• Soft Towels and Washcloths: Special hooded towels help keep babies warm after bathing.

6. Health and safety

• Digital Thermometer: Essential for checking a baby's temperature

• Baby Nail Clippers or Scissors: Baby nails grow astonishingly rapidly!

• Nasal Aspirator: For cleansing the baby's small nostrils

• Outlet Covers and Other Baby-proofing Items: As newborns develop, they explore, making baby-proofing important.

7. On-the-Go Essentials
• Infant Car Seat: A non-negotiable necessity for transporting infants home from the hospital
• Stroller: Depending on your preferences, there are numerous varieties, from jogging to lightweight alternatives.
• Baby carrier or sling: offers a hands-free option to keep the baby near.

8. Soothing and entertainment
• Pacifiers: Some newborns turn to these for comfort.
• Toys: soft, baby-safe toys for stimulation and teething
• Swing or bouncer: great equipment to calm and amuse infants.

While every baby and family is different, and what's necessary for one can be optional for another, this list covers the key essentials that most infants and their parents will require. Always examine your individual requirements and circumstances, and don't hesitate to ask for opinions from friends, family, or physicians.

CHAPTER 8: RELATIONSHIPS AND SUPPORT

Welcoming a new baby is a dramatic life transition that impacts not just parents but also the whole network of connections around them. The need for understanding, patience, and persistent support is vital during this transforming period. Here's an examination of how relationships form and the value of support systems:

1. The Parental Relationship:

• New Roles: Transitioning to parenting may transform identities. Open discussion about duties, obligations, and emotions may reinforce the partnership.

• Emotional Changes: Hormonal imbalances and sleep deprivation may heighten emotions. Recognizing these shifts might assist in being patient and understanding with one another.

• Intimacy: The dynamic of closeness typically alters after a pregnancy. While physical intimacy could be reduced briefly, emotional closeness might grow.

• Time Management: Balancing infant care, personal time, and couple time demands careful preparation. Regularly organizing date nights or shared activities might help sustain the relationship's vibrancy.

2. Extended Family:

• Grandparents: They may be wonderful sources of knowledge and aid, but they could also have strong ideas about child rearing. Setting limits while understanding their experience is vital.

• Siblings: The arrival of a new baby might provoke sentiments of enthusiasm, jealousy, or insecurity among older siblings. Reassuring them and including them in newborn care helps ease the adjustment.

3. Friends:

• Childless Friends: The dynamics may vary, particularly if they're at various life stages. Maintaining these connections requires mutual understanding and effort.

• New Parent Friends: Connecting with other parents may provide mutual support, understanding, and chances for socialization where infants are welcome.

4. Professional Support

• Medical Professionals: Regular check-ins with pediatricians and obstetricians/gynecologists assure the well-being of both baby and mother.

• Lactation Consultants: If breastfeeding, these specialists may provide important information and solutions to issues.

• Mental Health Professionals: Postpartum sadness or anxiety affects many new parents. Therapists or counselors may provide coping skills and assistance.

5. Community and Groups:

• Parenting Groups: These are places to share experiences, ask questions, and interact with parents in similar circumstances.

• Online Communities: Digital platforms may be a 24/7 resource for guidance, sharing, and support.

6. Self-Support:

• Self-care: Parents should also emphasize their well-being. Simple activities like reading, brief walks, or hobbies may refresh the mind and body.

• Open Communication: Sharing sentiments, worries, or pleasures may minimize feelings of isolation and develop better ties with loved ones.

Key Takeaways

The postpartum phase is commonly nicknamed the "fourth trimester" because of its importance. As relationships change and adjust to the new addition, the necessity of a robust support system can't be stressed enough. It really takes a village to raise a kid, and creating this feeling of camaraderie and understanding helps not only the newborn but the whole family.

A. Nurturing Your Relationship

In the frenzy of life's duties, particularly with the addition of children, sustaining your love connection may often take a backseat. However, sustaining a strong relationship is vital to general well-being and pleasure. Here's some advice on how to establish and nurture the link with your significant other:

1. Prioritize quality time

• Date Nights: Whether it's a nice dinner out or a movie night in, routinely committing time solely to each other may renew passion.
• Shared Activities: Engaging in shared interests or trying out new things together may deepen your friendship.

2. Communicate openly

• Active Listening: Listen to comprehend, not only to answer. This tells your lover that they're cherished.
• Express Yourself: Be upfront about your emotions, worries, and wants, promoting two-way communication.
• Avoid the blame game: use "I feel" phrases instead of pointing fingers.

3. Show Appreciation

• Little Gestures: Small gestures like leaving love notes or cooking a surprise dinner may make a major impact.
• Say 'Thank You: Regularly express thanks for the simple things your spouse does.

4. Keep the spark alive

• Physical Intimacy: This isn't only about sex; it's also about holding hands, embracing, or just touching. Physical connection develops emotional connectedness.

• Surprises: Spontaneous actions or surprises, like organizing a spontaneous retreat, may renew romance.

5. Manage conflicts constructively

• Stay calm. Avoid raising your voice or allowing emotions to take control completely.

Seek Understanding: Aim to comprehend your partner's viewpoint instead of winning an argument.

• Take breaks: If things become too hot, it's appropriate to take a pause and continue the issue later.

6. Set Boundaries

• Personal Space: Respect the need for individual space and time. Everyone needs times of isolation or time with their own friends.

• Digital Detox: Allocate times when phones, TVs, and other displays are off and focused only on each other.

7. Plan for the Future

• Discuss Objectives: Regularly speak about your common objectives and individual ambitions.

• Work as a Team: Approach life's obstacles and ambitions as a unified front.

8. Seek external support.

• Couples therapy: There's no shame in seeking expert help. A relationship specialist may give you tools and tactics to improve your partnership.

• Spend time with other couples: Being among peers who are also in good relationships may be inspiring and bring fresh ideas.

9. Remember the Basics

• Trust and honesty are the cornerstones of every enduring partnership.

• Shared principles: Regularly examine and discuss the basic principles that brought you together.

10. Continue growing together.
• Educate yourself: Attend courses or study books on boosting partnerships.
• Adapt and evolve: Change is inevitable. Embrace it and develop together.

In essence, developing a relationship is a continual process that involves work, understanding, and mutual respect. Amidst the bustle of everyday life, making your relationship a priority will guarantee it not only survives but flourishes.

B. Seeking Help from Friends and Family

In life's varied path, there are instances when seeking support, understanding, or even just a listening ear from friends and family is crucial.

Here's how to properly contact and accept help from your loved ones:

1. Recognize the need for help.
• Self-Awareness It's crucial to recognize and accept when you're feeling overwhelmed, frightened, or unable to manage events on your own.

2. Be specific in your request.
• Explicit Needs: Instead of making generic remarks like "I'm so stressed," describe your needs, "Can you help watch the kids on Friday evening?"
• Task-oriented Assistance: If you need assistance with duties, like moving houses or arranging an event, lay them out so it's easier for others to see where they can assist.

3. Choose the Right Person:
• Strengths and Skills: Approach people based on their talents or knowledge connected to your demand.

• Emotional Capacity: Consider the emotional availability of the individual. It's crucial to seek help from someone who isn't already overloaded with their own issues.

4. Create a safe space.

• Open Communication: Ensure the climate is favorable for open, honest talks without fear of judgment.

• Confidentiality: If the subject is private, reassure them of your need for confidentiality and ask if they're okay with keeping the chat discreet.

5. Be open to comments.

• Active Listening: While the main purpose may be to seek help, it's equally useful to listen to any comments or advice.

• Respect differing perspectives: Your friends and relatives could have different perspectives. While you don't have to agree, respect their opinion.

6. Offer reciprocity.

• Gratitude: Always show your thanks for their aid or understanding, whether via words, a thank-you letter, or gestures.

• Reciprocal Support: Let them know you're there for them too. Relationships flourish with reciprocal support.

7. Understand Boundaries

• Respect limitations: Everyone has their limitations. If someone is unable to help, understand and appreciate their reasons.

• Avoid overburdening: Continually depending on the same person might strain the connection. It's vital to broaden your support system.

8. Seek group support.

• Support Groups: Sometimes, it's good to include a group, like holding a gathering where friends and family may join together to assist with a certain activity or event.

• Shared Experiences: Engaging many people might be particularly beneficial if they've gone through comparable situations.

9. Stay Transparent

• Honest Conversations: If sentiments shift or if you're feeling more supported or overwhelmed, discuss these feelings to guarantee clarity.

10. Nurture the relationship.

• Beyond the Request: Regularly communicate with friends and family outside of times of need. It's crucial to preserve and cultivate these ties.

Remember, requesting assistance is a show of strength, not weakness. In times of vulnerability, ties with friends and family may provide unequaled support, understanding, and love. But it's equally crucial to give back, ensuring these partnerships stay balanced and healthy.

CHAPTER 9: UNDERSTANDING LABOUR AND DELIVERY

Labor and delivery signify the climax of pregnancy, culminating in the birth of a baby. This procedure, although normal and common, is complicated and differs for each woman. Here's a complete outline to help expecting moms and their partners realize what to anticipate:

1. Pre-labor signs:

• Lightening: This refers to the baby "dropping" or resting lower into the pelvis.

• Braxton Hicks Contractions: These "false" contractions are intermittent and typically not painful, helping to prepare the uterus.

• Loss of the Mucus Plug: This gelatinous plug, which closes the cervix, could be evacuated days or hours before labor occurs.

• Water Breaking: The rupture of the amniotic sac might result in a trickle or gush of fluid.

2. The Stages of Labor:

• First Stage (Cervical Changes): The cervix dilated and effaced (thins out). This stage comprises three stages: early labor, active labor, and transition.

• Second Stage (Delivery): Begin when the cervix is completely dilated and finish with the baby's delivery.

• Third Stage (afterbirth): The placenta and fetal membranes are evacuated.

3. Variations in Labor Patterns

• Prodromal Labor: Contractions start and cease for hours or even days before active labor starts.

• Back Labor: Pain is felt mostly in the lower back, generally because of the baby's position.

• Rapid Labor: Labor and delivery occur in only a few hours.

4. Methods of Delivery

• Vaginal birth: natural delivery via the birth canal

• Cesarean Section (C-section): A surgical technique where the infant is delivered via incisions in the abdomen and uterus

• VBAC (Vaginal Birth After Cesarean): Attempting a vaginal birth after a prior C-section

5. Pain Management Options

• Natural Methods: Breathing methods, exercise, warm baths, and massage

• Drugs: Epidurals, spinal blocks, and pain-relief drugs

6. Possible Interventions

• Induction: initiating labor by means like breaking the water or utilizing drugs like Pitocin
• Assisted Delivery: Using equipment such as forceps or a vacuum extractor to help deliver the baby

7. Post-delivery

• Initial Assessments: The Apgar score analyzes the baby's health at one and five minutes following delivery.
• Skin-to-Skin Contact: Immediate contact helps in bonding, breastfeeding, and stabilizing the baby's temperature.
• Delayed cord clamping: Waiting to cut the umbilical cord may have advantages for the newborn, including increased blood volume.

8. Potential difficulties

• While most births are easy, it's crucial to identify potential difficulties like:
• Prolonged labor: labor that lasts longer than intended.
• Breech Position: The infant is positioned feet or buttocks first.

• Placental issues: Such as placenta previa (covering the cervix) or placental abruption (detaching early).

Understanding the subtleties of labor and delivery may provide pregnant parents with the information they need to make educated choices, relieve concerns, and facilitate a smoother birthing journey. It's vital to speak with healthcare professionals, ask questions, and voice preferences or concerns.

A. Stages of Labor

Labor is a complicated procedure that leads to the delivery of a baby. It's often separated into three primary phases, each distinguished by unique occurrences and various lengths. Understanding these phases may help pregnant moms and their partners know what to anticipate throughout the childbirth process.

1. First Stage: Dilation and Effacement of the Cervix

This stage is the longest and consists of three phases:

Early labor (latent phase)
• Cervical Dilation: The cervical cavity dilates up to 3 cm.
• Contractions: mild, irregular contractions that progressively become more regular and stronger.
• Duration: This may take many hours, particularly for first-time moms.
• Signs: Mild back discomfort, cramping, and the production of a mucus plug (occasionally tinged with blood).

Active Labor:
• Cervical Dilation: The cervical cavity dilates from 4 cm to 7 cm.
• Contractions: more regular, frequent, and powerful, lasting around 45–60 seconds each.
• Duration: Typically lasts 3-5 hours.
• Signs: increased pain, harder contractions, and the impulse to move or change positions

Transition Phase:

• Cervical Dilation: The cervical dilation ranges from 8 cm to 10 cm.

•Contractions: Extremely forceful, lasting 60–90 seconds with a brief pause in between.

• Duration: Shortest period, lasting anything from a few minutes to a couple of hours.

• Signs: increased intensity, sensations of pressure, potential nausea, and the impulse to push

2. Second Stage: Pushing and Birth

• Cervical Dilation: The cervix is completely dilated at 10 cm.

• Contractions: They continue but may spread out, giving the mother a little respite.

• Duration: Lasts from 20 minutes to 2 hours.

• Process: With each contraction, the woman pushes, helping the baby descend down the delivery canal. This period ends with the birth of the baby.

• Signs: intense need to push, straining, and burning sensations as the baby crowns

3. Third Stage: Delivery of the Placenta

• Process: After the baby is delivered, the uterus continues to contract to evacuate the placenta.

• Duration: It usually takes 5 to 30 minutes post-birth.

• Signs: Mild contractions persist until the placenta is delivered. There can be a sense of fullness and the need to push again.

• Importance: It's vital for healthcare practitioners to ensure the complete placenta is ejected to avoid problems.

Understanding these phases and their possible differences might reduce some of the anxiety connected with labor. It's also essential for birthing partners to be conversant with these phases to provide adequate assistance. Always interact with healthcare personnel throughout labor to ask questions, understand progress, and receive assistance.

B. Delivery Methods and Complications

Childbirth is a unique experience for every woman, and although many births progress without difficulties, it's crucial to be aware of the different delivery procedures and the concerns that might develop.

Delivery Methods

1. Vaginal Birth:
• A natural method when the baby is born via the birth canal;
• Can entail several positions: reclining on the back, squatting, or on hands and knees.
• Recovery time is often shorter compared to a C-section.

2. Cesarean Section (C-section):
• A surgical surgery when the baby is delivered via an incision in the mother's belly and uterus.
• Often planned ahead for different medical reasons, but may also be an emergency choice depending on difficulties during labor.

• Recovery is prolonged and may need additional pain treatment.

3. VBAC (Vaginal Birth After Cesarean):
• A vaginal birth attempted by a woman who has previously undergone a C-section;
• Not all women are eligible for VBAC, and it comes with special risks, like uterine rupture.

4. Water Birth:
• The procedure of giving birth in a tub of warm water is thought to be less stressful for the infant and less difficult for the mother.
• Not all women are candidates, and there are benefits and downsides to consider.

5. Assisted Vaginal Delivery:
• Instruments, such as forceps or a vacuum, are used to assist the baby out of the delivery canal.
• This is usually considered if the infant is displaying indications of discomfort or the mother is fatigued.

Complications during delivery:

1. Prolonged Labor (Failure to Progress):
• Labor is exceptionally protracted, or contractions are not effective in opening the cervix.
• Causes might include a huge baby, a narrow pelvis, or inadequate contractions.

2. Perineal Tears:
• Tears in the tissue between the vaginal entrance and the anus They vary in severity and may need sutures.

3. Umbilical Cord Issues:
• Cord Prolapse: The chord descends through the cervix before the infant. A medical emergency.
• Cord compression: The chord gets compressed, often owing to the infant's position, decreasing blood supply to the newborn.

4. Placental Abruption:
• The placenta detaches from the uterine wall before childbirth, which might deprive the infant of oxygen and nourishment.

5. Breech Birth:
• The infant is positioned feet or buttocks first instead of head-down. It might result in additional problems during vaginal birth.

6. Shoulder dystocia:
• The baby's head goes through the birth canal, but the shoulders get trapped. This may be harmful for both mother and baby.

7. Postpartum hemorrhage:
• heavy bleeding after birth, which may be life-threatening.

8. Uterine Rupture:
• A rip in the uterus, especially frequent in women who have undergone a past C-section.

9. Amniotic Fluid Embolism:
• Amniotic fluid enters the mother's circulation, leading to life-threatening problems.

Every woman's experience during delivery will be different. While issues might emerge, many are controllable with quick and adequate medical treatment. It's vital for pregnant moms to keep regular prenatal check-ups, interact with their healthcare professionals, and educate themselves to make educated choices throughout labor and delivery.

CHAPTER 10: THE FIRST WEEKS WITH YOUR BABY

The first few weeks following bringing your newborn home are a combination of pleasure, hardship, and new experiences. You're getting to know your tiny one while navigating the intricacies of postpartum recovery. Here's an insight into what you might anticipate and ideas for managing this lovely but intense period:

1. Feeding Your Baby:

• Breastfeeding: it may take time for both mother and baby to get the hang of breastfeeding. Latch difficulties, engorgement, and nipple pain are typical. Lactation consultants may be a great resource.

• Formula Feeding: If you elect for or need to use formula, ensure you're using the right measurements and following cleanliness measures.

2. Diapering:

• Frequent Changes: Newborns have frequent bowel motions. Keeping them clean and dry minimizes diaper rash.
• Umbilical Cord Care: Until the stump comes out, tuck the diaper underneath it and ensure the region is clean and dry.

3. Sleep Patterns:

• Erratic Sleep: Newborns sleep a lot but in short spurts, frequently waking up every 2-3 hours to feed.
• Safe Sleep Practices: Place the baby on their back in a crib or cot without pillows, blankets, or toys.

4. Baby's Health Checkups:

• First Doctor's Visit: Typically arranged within the first week to evaluate weight, height, and overall well-being.
• Indicators of illness: Be vigilant for indicators like fever, tiredness, or trouble breathing and visit your physician.

5. Postpartum Recovery:

• Physical Healing: Whether you had a vaginal delivery or a C-section, your body needs time to recover. Expect vaginal discharge (lochia), discomfort, and contractions.
• Emotional well-being: hormonal fluctuations might contribute to the "baby blues" or more serious postpartum depression. Open communication and seeking assistance if required are key.

6. Bonding with Your Baby:

• Skin-to-Skin Contact: This improves bonding, relaxes the infant, and has several health advantages.
• Talking and singing: These interactions are important for your baby's cognitive and emotional development.

7. Caring for Yourself:

• Rest When Possible: Sleep when the baby naps, and don't hesitate to ask for assistance.
• Nutrition: Eating balanced meals improves

healing and offers energy.

• Stay hydrated. This is particularly vital if you're nursing.

8. Seeking Support:

• Family and friends: They may give emotional support, assist with housework, or simply provide companionship.
• Support groups: Connecting with other new parents may be soothing and educational.

9. Trusting Your Instincts:

• Parental Intuition: Trust your gut feelings about your baby's requirements and your well-being.
• Keep educated: While intuition is significant, it's equally necessary to keep educated via trustworthy sources and guidance from healthcare specialists.

10. Remember, it's a phase:

• Challenging Moments: There will be challenging moments, but they are fleeting.
• Cherish the Moments: Amidst the hardships,

there will be innumerable joyful moments. Take the time to appreciate and record them.

The early weeks with your infant are a remarkable voyage of love, learning, and adaptability. While it's normal to feel overwhelmed, realize that every hurdle encountered is a step ahead in the amazing path of motherhood. Seeking aid, practicing self-care, and celebrating tiny achievements may make this phase more comfortable and pleasant.

A. Bringing Baby Home

The moment you've excitedly anticipated is finally here: taking your baby home. While it's a moment filled with pleasure and excitement, it's also a new chapter loaded with difficulties and lessons. Here's what you need to know and consider while introducing your kid to their new environment:

1. The Car Ride Home:

• Car Seat: Ensure you have a rear-facing car seat correctly placed. Many hospitals won't let you leave without one. Familiarize yourself with its functioning before the baby comes.

2. Setting Up a Safe Environment:

• Resting environment: The infant should have a secure, clutter-free resting environment, preferably a crib or cot with a firm mattress.

• Pet Introduction: If you have pets, expose them to the baby's smell first and monitor their first encounter.

• Temperature: Maintain a suitable indoor temperature, neither too hot nor too cold.

3. Daily Routines:

• Feeding: Whether you're breastfeeding or formula-feeding, arrange a peaceful and comfortable area for feedings.

• Diapering: Have a distinct changing room equipped with diapers, wipes, and creams.

• Bathing: In the earliest weeks, sponge baths are advised until the umbilical cord comes off.

4. Visitors and Hygiene:

• Limit visitors: The baby's immune system is still growing. It's appropriate to restrict visits during the first several weeks.

• Hygiene: Ensure visitors wash their hands before touching the infant. Avoid exposure to ill people.

5. Bonding Time:

• Skin-to-skin: This technique fosters bonding, maintains the baby's temperature, and may even boost nursing success.

• Talk and sing: Even if the infant doesn't comprehend words, the sound of your voice is comforting and helps auditory development.

6. Monitor the baby's health:

• Signs of Illness: Look out for signs including unusual tiredness, fever, difficulties feeding, or continuous crying. Don't hesitate to visit your doctor.

• Regular Checkups: Attend all planned pediatric checkups to verify the baby's development and health are on track.

7. Take Care of Yourself:

• Rest: Sleep may be elusive with a baby. Sleep when the baby naps, and don't hesitate to ask for assistance when required.

• Nutrition: A healthy diet is vital, particularly while nursing.

• Mental well-being: It's normal to feel stressed. Speak about your thoughts, and consider attending a support group for new parents.

8. Establishing Routines:

• Consistent Patterns: Over time, strive to create consistent eating, bathing, and sleeping patterns. It makes the infant feel safe and may enhance sleep habits.

9. Documenting Milestones

• Capture Moments: Time flies! Take photographs, record milestones, and consider starting a baby book.

10. Seeking Support and Resources:

• Pediatrician: They are your go-to for any worries concerning the baby's health.

• Lactation Consultants: If you're encountering issues with nursing, they provide essential insights and answers.

• Parenting groups: connecting with other parents may provide emotional support and practical assistance.

Bringing your kid home is a huge event, loaded with a combination of emotions. It's a voyage of love, patience, and progress. While it's crucial to protect your baby's comfort and safety, remember to also care for yourself. The foundations set in these first weeks may pave the way for a satisfying parenting experience.

B. Postpartum Care for Mom

The postpartum period, commonly referred to as the "fourth trimester," is an important phase after delivery. While considerable care is devoted to the infant, the mother's physical and emotional recovery is equally vital. Here's a detailed resource on postpartum care for the new mother:

1. Physical Recovery:
• Vaginal Birth Recovery: Expect vaginal pain, particularly if you received sutures for perineal rips. Sit on a comfy couch, try cold packs, and consider sitz baths for relief.
• C-section recovery: keep the wound clean and dry. Avoid hard lifting and monitor for symptoms of infection, including increasing redness or leaking.
• Lochia (postpartum bleeding): This is a natural vaginal discharge that's first bloody, eventually becoming lighter in color and flow. Use maternity pads, not tampons.

2. Breast Care:

• Engorgement: Breasts may grow big, hard, and painful when they begin producing milk. Frequent feeding or pumping and cold compresses may assist.

• Nipple Care: Nipples could become damaged or painful. Using lanolin lotion and keeping a healthy latch when nursing may help avoid or reduce this.

3. Bowel and Bladder Functions:

• Constipation: This is common post-delivery. Drinking water, ingesting fiber-rich meals, and taking moderate stool softeners may assist.

• Hemorrhoids: Use over-the-counter lotions or witch hazel pads for relief.

• Urinary incontinence: Kegel exercises help strengthen pelvic muscles and improve control.

4. Emotional Well-Being:

• Baby Blues: Many women suffer mood fluctuations, sorrow, and irritability immediately after delivering. This normally resolves after a week or two.

• Postpartum Depression (PPD): More severe than the baby blues, PPD is characterized by extended emotions of sorrow, worry, and despair. Seek expert treatment if you suspect PPD.

5. Hormonal Changes:

• Night Sweats: Hormonal fluctuations might cause excessive sweating. Sleeping in a cool environment and wearing breathable textiles may assist.
• Hair Loss: Temporary hair loss postpartum is usual due to altered hormone levels.

6. Birth Control and Intimacy:

• Contraception: Discuss birth control choices with your healthcare professional, particularly because certain methods might influence nursing.
• Resuming Intercourse: Wait until you feel physically and emotionally ready. Initial postpartum sex might be unpleasant; use lubricant and a soft position.

7. Fitness and Diet:

• Gentle Exercise: Begin with mild workouts like walking and gradually work your way up, securing your doctor's approval.

• Diet: A balanced diet improves recuperation and encourages breastfeeding. Stay hydrated and select meals high in iron and protein.

8. Self-care:

• Rest: Sleep while the baby naps. Fatigue may increase emotional issues.

• Time for Yourself: Allocate minutes for self-care, whether reading, bathing, or other relaxing practices.

9. Seeking Support:

• Healthcare Provider: Regular postpartum check-ups ensure you're recovering well and offer a chance to address issues.

• Support groups: Connecting with other new moms may be soothing and informative.

10. Communicate with your partner:

• Share Feelings: Discuss physical and emotional changes, and remember that they too can be navigating new problems and feelings.

The postpartum period is a time of great adjustment and recovery. While catering to the baby's demands, new moms should remember to prioritize their well-being, requesting assistance when required. Proper postpartum care builds the framework for an easier transition into parenthood and ensures the health and happiness of both mother and baby.

CHAPTER 11: PARENTING 101

Parenting, frequently called the most hard but rewarding profession, doesn't come with a comprehensive guidebook. It's a path of ongoing learning, adaptation, and progress. As you begin your journey, here's a primer to take you through the fundamentals of parenting:

1. Bonding and Attachment:
• Early Days: Skin-to-skin contact, nursing, and just holding your infant may establish a profound emotional bond.
• Consistent Care: Responding immediately to your baby's needs, particularly in the early months, develops security and confidence.

2. Effective Communication:
• Active Listening: Pay attention to both verbal and non-verbal clues from your kid.

• Age-appropriate Conversations: Adjust the complexity of topics depending on your child's age and knowledge.

3. Consistency is key:
• Routine: Children thrive on predictability. Regular habits for eating, sleeping, and playing give stability.
• Discipline: Set explicit expectations and penalties, ensuring that they're enforced consistently.

4. Lead by example:
• Model Behavior: Children are good observers. Demonstrate ideals and actions you would like others to acquire.
• Admit Mistakes: Teach humility and responsibility by acknowledging when you're incorrect and apologizing.

5. Foster Independence:
• Teach responsibility: assign age-appropriate duties and responsibilities.

• Decision-making: Allow children to make decisions, helping them comprehend consequences and learn from experiences.

6. Encourage learning and curiosity:
• Educational Play: Opt for toys and activities that develop their thinking.
• Ask Questions: Encourage children to investigate the world around them and seek answers.

7. Set Boundaries:
• Clear restrictions: Set clear and fair restrictions, stating the reasoning behind them.
• Positive Reinforcement: Praise excellent conduct, which frequently works better than penalizing disobedience.

8. Build resilience:
• Problem-solving: Instead of instantly fixing everything for them, help them discover solutions.

• Face Challenges: Support them through failures and disappointments, teaching tenacity and resilience.

9. Physical and emotional health:

• Balanced diet and exercise: promote healthy eating habits and frequent physical exercise.
• Emotional Expression: Create a place where kids may express emotions without judgment.

10. Stay updated and seek support:

• Continuous Learning: Parenting Changes Stay current with books, seminars, or courses.
• Build a Support System: Surround yourself with a network of family, friends, or parent groups for guidance and support.

Parenting 101 is not about perfection but about understanding, love, patience, and guidance. Each kid is unique, forcing you to adapt and develop with them. Remember, although there could be various parenting approaches and ideologies, your intuition, paired with love, will frequently guide you in the correct direction.

A. The Joys and Challenges of Parenthood

Embarking on the adventure of motherhood is analogous to sailing a wide sea filled with times of peaceful tranquility and tumultuous storms. It's a life-altering adventure packed with highs and lows, pleasures and hardships. Let's go into the core of this remarkable experience:

The Joys of Parenthood:

1. Firsts and Milestones: From the baby's first grin, walk, and word to later life milestones like graduations and marriages, these events fill parents with pride and satisfaction.

2. Unconditional Love: The profound, unexplainable link and love experienced with a

kid is one of the purest and most fulfilling sensations.

3. Personal Growth: Parenthood frequently brings forth qualities like patience and resilience you never thought you possessed.

4. Rediscovery: Viewing the world through your child's eyes rekindles surprise and desire for life's basic joys.

5. Legacy and Lessons: Passing on knowledge, values, and life lessons to the next generation offers a tremendous sense of purpose.

6. Companionship: Having a kid means having a lifetime companion, someone to share events, memories, and experiences with.

Challenges of Parenthood:

1. Sleep deprivation: Especially in the early stages, restless nights may take a toll on physical and emotional well-being.

2. Financial Strain: Raising a kid may be costly, with expenditures from daycare through school and beyond.

3. Balancing Act: Juggling work, personal time, relationships, and child-rearing may become difficult.

4. Emotional Stress: From worry about your child's well-being to negotiating the complexity of their teenage years, emotional obstacles are plentiful.

5. Differences in Parenting Styles: Partners could have diverse views and approaches to parenting, resulting in disagreements.

6. Letting Go: As children grow and seek independence, parents typically battle with the problem of letting go, from the first day of school to when they leave the nest.

7. Self-disregard: In the maelstrom of parenting a kid, parents frequently disregard their own needs, health, and goals.

Finding Balance:

1. Support Systems: Building and depending on a support network, whether it is family, friends, or support groups, may ease many issues.

2. Open Communication: Regularly sharing emotions, anxieties, and expectations with your spouse and even with your kid may create understanding and identify solutions.

3. Self-care: Prioritizing self-care, both physically and emotionally, is not selfish. It guarantees you're at your best for your kid.

4. Stay informed: Parenting books, courses, and programs may give important insights and coping skills.

5. Celebrate the modest moments: Amidst the hardships, it's crucial to embrace the modest, daily delights that motherhood delivers.

Parenthood, although certainly tough, has immense benefits. Embracing all the pleasures and hardships with patience, compassion, and love makes the trip all the more enjoyable.

B. Creating a Strong Parenting Foundation

Building a firm foundation for parenting is analogous to constructing the framework for a home that must survive many storms and change through time. It's about fostering an atmosphere of trust, understanding, and consistency. Here's a guide to help you develop a healthy parenting foundation:

1. Communication is key:

• Open Dialogues: Foster an atmosphere where children feel they can speak about anything, no matter how large or small.

• Active Listening: Truly listen to your children's worries, emotions, and questions without quick judgment.

2. Consistency and boundaries:

• Stability: Kids thrive in a steady environment. Regular schedules for meals, schoolwork, and sleep may create a feeling of stability.

• Set clear limits: While it's good to be flexible sometimes, consistent limits help youngsters learn expectations and consequences.

3. Lead by example:

• Model Behavior: Children frequently mimic adults. Display the values, manners, and conduct you would like them to embrace.

• Admit Mistakes: Showing that you're not perfect teaches kids humility and the value of accepting responsibility.

4. Quality Time:

• Shared things: Engage in things that you both like, from reading together to outdoor trips.

• Stay Present: In the era of distractions, ensure you're mentally present throughout your time together.

5. Educate and guide:

• Teachable Moments: Use ordinary circumstances to deliver lessons about values, decision-making, and life skills.

• Encourage Curiosity: Support their drive for knowledge by answering questions, exploring together, or introducing them to resources.

6. Emotional Intelligence:

• Express Feelings: Encourage unrestricted expression of feelings. Let them know it's alright to feel angry, sad, or puzzled, but it's crucial to handle these emotions wisely.

• Empathy: Teach children to understand and respect others' emotions.

7. Foster Independence:

• Age-appropriate Chores: Assign duties like cleaning up their room or assisting with dishes to develop responsibility.

• Decision-making: Allow children to make decisions (within limits), emphasizing the awareness of consequences.

8. Discipline with Love

• Constructive Feedback: Instead of simply punishing them, concentrate on teaching them what they can do better next time.

• Avoid Negative Labels: Refrain from using negative labels or name-calling, concentrating instead on the behavior, not the kid.

9. Build resilience:

• Overcoming Challenges: Instead of protecting them from every impediment, help them confront problems and learn from setbacks.

• Problem-solving: Encourage children to think through solutions to issues they meet.

10. Stay informed and adapt.

• Parenting Resources: Books, conferences, and parenting groups provide ideas that may aid in overcoming different issues.

•   Flexibility: As   children   grow,   their requirements vary. Stay adaptive, re-evaluating techniques and routines as required.

Creating a good parental foundation doesn't entail perfection. It's about creating a friendship built on trust, respect, and understanding. With this foundation, you'll be better able to face the ever-evolving difficulties and pleasures of motherhood, leading your kid along life's path with love and knowledge.

CHAPTER 12: LOOKING AHEAD

Looking Ahead encompasses the proactive attitude of expecting and planning for the plethora of changes, difficulties, and pleasures that come with pregnancy and the ensuing journey of motherhood. As we travel the road of life, the horizon ahead is frequently filled with doubts, ambitions, and boundless possibilities. Whether in the context of personal development, parenting, profession, or relationships, looking forward is about anticipating the future, creating objectives, and preparing for what's to come. Here's a strategy to help you stare ahead with clarity and purpose:

1. Anticipating Physical and Emotional Changes: Pregnancy brings about a surge of modifications in a woman's body and mentality. Looking forward involves comprehending these transformations and preparing intellectually, emotionally, and physically for them.

2. Preparation for delivery: From deciding between hospital or home delivery to comprehending different pain management choices, thinking ahead requires making educated decisions regarding the birthing process.

3. Postpartum and Beyond: The postpartum phase may be as stressful as the pregnancy itself. Anticipating probable problems like postpartum depression, breastfeeding difficulty, or sleep disruptions helps make this transition simpler.

4. Financial and logistical planning: The addition of a new family member typically requires budgetary modifications. This can entail planning for medical expenditures, setting up a nursery, or even long-term preparations like college funds.

5. Relationship Dynamics: The presence of a child may substantially affect the dynamics of a partnership. Couples may plan ahead by discussing honestly about probable pressures, sharing duties, and developing their relationship.

6. Future Parenthood Challenges: Beyond the earliest phases, planning forward also means thinking about the probable problems of having a kid, from toddler tantrums to adolescent rebellions.

7. Building a Help System: Anticipating the need for help, whether from family, friends, or professional services, ensures that parents have the essential assistance when needed.

8. Personal Growth and Self-Care: Amidst the demands of parenthood, people shouldn't overlook their well-being. Looking forward can require carving out personal time or organizing date nights to preserve balance.

Looking forward is more than simply preparing for the future. It's about thinking big, creating goals, and matching actions with those visions. While the way ahead could be riddled with unknowns, it's the preparation, tenacity, and enthusiasm that determine the journey's depth and satisfaction. Whatever is ahead, approach it with hope, preparedness, and an unshakeable spirit.

A. Balancing Work and Family

In today's fast-paced world, maintaining a balance between professional commitments and family life is a difficulty many encounter. Both need time, focus, and energy. Yet establishing this balance is vital for personal well-being, career success, and family peace. Here's a guide to help you handle the delicate dance between work and family:

1. Set clear priorities:
Identify Key Goals: Determine what's most essential in both your work and personal lives.
Assign Time: Based on these priorities, assign time to key activities and obligations in both sectors.

2. Effective Time Management:

Plan ahead: Use calendars or planners to set out job tasks, family activities, and personal obligations.

Avoid Procrastination: Tackling duties immediately helps minimize last-minute rushes that interfere with family time.

3. Set Boundaries:

Work Hours: Stick to established work hours as precisely as possible. Avoid taking work home routinely.

Digital Detox: Allocate periods when gadgets are put away, concentrating completely on family.

4. Quality Over Quantity:

Engaged Family Time: Make sure the time spent with family is meaningful. Engage in activities that build connections.

Mindful Work: When at work, be totally present and productive to guarantee efficiency.

5. Flexibility is key:

Flexible Work Hours: If feasible, arrange flexible hours or remote work days to meet family demands.

Go with the flow. Sometimes, despite preparation, things go astray. Adaptability may alleviate stress in such scenarios.

6. Share responsibilities:

Delegate jobs: At work, delegate jobs when feasible. At home, allocate responsibilities among family members.

Team Approach: Foster a spirit of collaboration in the family where everyone contributes and supports one another.

7. Self-care and personal time:

Prioritize Yourself: Regularly schedule time for things you enjoy, whether it's reading, hobbies, or leisure.

Stay healthy: Regular exercise, a balanced diet, and enough sleep guarantee you have the energy for both work and family.

8. Open Communication:

Address calendars: Regularly address job responsibilities and family calendars to ensure everyone is in the know.

Express Feelings: Talk about problems, pressures, and triumphs in both work and home contexts with your spouse or family.

9. Seek External Support:

Daycare: Reliable daycare may reduce work-related stressors and guarantee your child's well-being.

Networking: Connect with people in similar circumstances for suggestions, support, and shared experiences.

10. Regularly evaluate and adjust:

Check-in with yourself: Periodically analyze how you feel about your work-family balance.

Make the necessary changes: Based on these thoughts, alter schedules, priorities, or approaches to best support your balance.

Balancing work and family is a continual process of juggling, adapting, and reevaluating. While it may seem tough, with conscious work, communication, and support, it's possible to have a rewarding profession and foster a flourishing family life. Remember, it's not about reaching a perfect balance but finding the one that brings harmony and satisfaction to your life.

B. Future Family Planning

Planning for the future of your family is a huge duty that takes vision, planning, and constant changes. Whether you're contemplating growing your family, insuring your children's education, or ensuring comfort throughout your elderly years, here's a guide to help you manage future family planning:

1. Family Expansion:

Size and spacing: Consider how many children you intend to have and the age gap between them.

Financial Implications: Understand the financial needs of having additional children, from healthcare to schooling and everyday costs.

2. Financial Security:

Budgeting: Regularly adjust your family budget to accommodate changing requirements and spending.

Savings and Investments: Start early with savings plans or investments to secure a solid financial future.

Emergency Fund: Always have funds allocated for unforeseen events, such as medical crises or job losses.

3. Education Planning:

Early Start: Begin investing for your children's education early, examining choices like education savings accounts or mutual funds.

Research Scholarships: Stay updated about scholarship options, which might ease some school expenditures.

4. Health and Insurance:

Regular check-ups: ensure family members get periodic health check-ups.
Health Insurance: Invest in comprehensive health insurance coverage that covers many possible demands.
Life Insurance: Consider insurance that can sustain your family financially in case of unanticipated catastrophes.

5. Housing and Living Conditions:

Future Needs: As your family expands, assess if your existing living environment can support such adjustments.
Location: Think about the proximity to schools, jobs, healthcare, and other vital facilities.

6. Career Planning:

Work-life balance: Seek career possibilities that connect with your family's needs and ideals.

Skills Development: Regularly upgrade your skills to guarantee job stability and the chance for development.

7. Retirement Planning:

Pension Plans: Contribute consistently to retirement accounts or pension plans.

Retirement Lifestyle: Consider the lifestyle you desire to enjoy during retirement and prepare appropriately.

8. Estate and Will Planning:

Legal Documentation: Draft a will to guarantee your assets are dispersed as per your preferences.

Guardianship: If you have small children, establish guardianship choices in your will.

9. Open Communication:

Discuss with spouse: Regularly discuss your family's future goals with your spouse to ensure both are on the same page.

Include youngsters: As they get older, include youngsters in talks about family objectives and choices, developing understanding and teamwork.

10. Stay informed and adapt

Stay Updated: Changes in the economy, school system, or employment market might impact future planning. Stay informed and adjust as required.

Re-evaluation: Periodically examine and revise your plans to ensure they correspond with your family's developing needs and aspirations.

Future family planning is a dynamic process that demands attention, consideration, and constant revisions. While it's hard to forecast every curve in the road, detailed preparation may offer a feeling of stability and direction. With careful consideration and proactive efforts, you may prepare the road for a better, more secure future for your family.

CONCLUSION

As we approach the culmination of "Expecting 101," it's apparent that the process of anticipating and accepting motherhood is a complicated tapestry of emotions, obstacles, and unsurpassed delights. Each chapter, each insight, tries to illustrate the multidimensional experience of bringing new life into the world.

The importance of this trip lies not simply in the bodily changes and preparations but in the deep transition people endure as they mature into parents. Parenthood doesn't come with a guidebook; it's a lifetime process of learning, adjusting, and evolving. Every kid is unique, and every parent's experience is different; however, there are universal truths and knowledge that may guide us.

"Looking Ahead" is a significant concept ringing throughout this voyage. By anticipating, planning, and adjusting, parents may manage the nuances of pregnancy and the obstacles of parenting a child with more confidence and clarity.

It's crucial to remember that although education and preparation are invaluable, so is following one's intuition, seeking help when required, and cherishing each moment. Parenthood is as much about the destination as it is about the trip. It's about the late-night lullabies, the first steps, the hardships conquered together, and the unconditional love shared.

As we end this course, our aim is that "Expecting 101" acts as a valued companion, bringing insights, comfort, and direction. May it join you throughout the lovely, changing trip of anticipating and motherhood, reminding you always of the pleasure, wonder, and love that are ahead.

A. Reflecting on Your Journey

As we bring this book to a conclusion, it's an opportunity to stop, breathe, and reflect back on the adventure we've done together. Every page flipped and every chapter looked into has been a mirror reflecting not only universal truths but also your personal experiences, feelings, and goals.

The journey of anticipating and parenting, as we've realized, is as much about contemplation as it is about preparedness. It's a journey where every twist and turn, every high and low, adds richness to the fabric of our lives. The hardships endured and the milestones celebrated have formed you, teaching resilience, patience, and the infinite depths of love.

Reflecting on this trip is vital. It's in these times of introspection that we discover clarity, appreciation, and a greater knowledge of ourselves and our loved ones. It helps us to treasure the past, learn from our blunders, and dream about the future with hope and enthusiasm.

Remember, no two trips are the same. While books like these provide insights and shared experiences, your journey is completely yours, molded by your decisions, experiences, and the love you share with your family.

In the silence of thought, may you discover a wellspring of pleasure, strength, and thankfulness. May you recognize that every stride, even the doubtful ones, has been a dance of development and discovery. As this chapter finishes, realize that your path is a continuing adventure of love, learning, and accepting the magnificent unpredictability of life.

May your reflections be your guiding star, illuminating the way ahead with wisdom, warmth, and wonder.

B. Embracing the Adventure Ahead

As we put down the last lines of this book, it's time to transfer our focus from the pages to the broad horizon that lies before us. The path of anticipating and motherhood isn't simply a chapter in life; it's an ever-evolving experience, replete with unexpected turns, deep discoveries, and times of pure, unadulterated delight.

While this book has offered tools, insights, and common experiences, the actual spirit of the trip comes from the undiscovered frontiers of your particular journey. It's about plunging headlong into the unknown, equipped with knowledge but open to wonder, and embracing each day with bravery, curiosity, and love.

The path ahead will definitely have its fair share of problems. There will be restless nights, times of uncertainty, and lessons learned the hard way. But interwoven with them will be the first chuckles, steps taken on unsteady feet, loving embraces, and many other moments that will be carved in your heart forever.

Embracing the experience involves appreciating both the highs and the lows. It's about knowing that obstacles are simply stepping stones, turning you into resilient, caring, and ever-growing people and parents.

As you go on, let this book be a beloved companion, a reminder of the power inside you, and the endless possibilities that lie ahead. But also rely on your gut, depend on loved ones, and take time to luxuriate in the present.

In conclusion, here's to you, courageous adventurers. Here's to the stories you'll tell, the joy you'll share, and the limitless love that will lead you. The adventure awaits, and what a magnificent one it promises to be! Embrace it with open arms, an open heart, and the spirit of exploration.